Dupuytren's Disease

Michael B. Gottschalk • Nina Suh
Eric R. Wagner
Editors

Dupuytren's Disease

Current and Emerging Techniques

Springer

Editors
Michael B. Gottschalk
Orthopedics and Spine Center
Emory Healthcare
Atlanta, GA, USA

Nina Suh
Orthopedics and Spine Center
Emory Healthcare
Atlanta, GA, USA

Eric R. Wagner
Orthopedics and Spine Center
Emory Healthcare
Atlanta, GA, USA

ISBN 978-3-031-85872-7 ISBN 978-3-031-85873-4 (eBook)
https://doi.org/10.1007/978-3-031-85873-4

This Springer imprint is published by the registered company Springer Nature Switzerland AG
The registered company address is: Gewerbestrasse 11, 6330 Cham, Switzerland

Contents

Contributors

Adil Shahzad Ahmed Joseph Barnhart Department of Orthopaedic Surgery, Baylor College of Medicine, Houston, TX, USA

Armin Badre Western Hand & Upper Limb Facility, St. Albert, AB, Canada

Kier M. Blevins Department of Orthopaedic Surgery, Emory University School of Medicine, Atlanta, GA, USA

Spencer B. Chambers Department of Plastic & Reconstructive Surgery. Roth|McFarlane Hand & Upper Limb Center, Western University, London, ON, Canada

Harvey Chim, MD Division of Plastic and Reconstructive Surgery, Louisiana State University Health Sciences Center, New Orleans, LA, USA

Margaux Danby University of Kentucky College of Medicine, Lexington, KY, USA

Joshua Gillis Division of Plastic Surgery, NL Health Services, Memorial University, St. John, NL, Canada

Alexander R. Graf Department of Orthopedic Surgery, Hand and Upper Extremity Division, Medical College of Wisconsin, Milwaukee, WI, USA

Reed Hoyer Indiana Hand to Shoulder Center, Indianapolis, IN, USA

Sanjeev Kakar Mayo Clinic, Rochester, MN, USA

Robin Kamal Department of Orthopedics, Stanford University, Stanford, CA, USA

Nathan Khabyeh-Hasbani Department of Orthopaedic Surgery, Montefiore Medical Center, Bronx, NY, USA

Christopher Klifto Duke University, Durham, NC, USA

Steven M. Koehler Department of Orthopaedic Surgery, Montefiore Medical Center, Bronx, NY, USA

Michael Lapner Western Hand & Upper Limb Facility, St. Albert, AB, Canada

Sasha G. Létourneau Division of Plastic and Reconstructive Surgery, Western University, London, ON, Canada

Yibo Li Western Hand & Upper Limb Facility, St. Albert, AB, Canada

Yusha Katie Liu Division of Plastic Surgery, Department of Surgery, University of Washington, Seattle, WA, USA

Osvaldo Conde Lorenzo San Juan Bautista School of Medicine, Caguas, Puerto Rico

Paul Marji, MD Division of Plastic and Reconstructive Surgery, University of Florida College of Medicine, Gainesville, FL, USA

Conner J. McMains Department of Plastic Surgery, Medical College of Wisconsin, Milwaukee, WI, USA

Eric Mitchell Division of Plastic Surgery, Western University, London, ON, Canada

Maureen O'Shaughnessy University of Kentucky College of Medicine, Lexington, KY, USA

Jeremy E. Raducha St Luke's University Health Network, Bethlehem, PA, USA

Marco Rizzo Department of Orthopedic Surgery, Mayo Clinic, Rochester, MN, USA

Christine V. Schaeffer University of Kentucky Plastic & Reconstructive Surgery, Lexington, KY, USA

Mark P. Smith Department of Orthopaedic Surgery, Indiana University School of Medicine, Indianapolis, IN, USA

Nina Suh Department of Orthopaedics, Emory University School of Medicine, Atlanta, GA, USA

Brianne J. Sullivan, MD Division of Plastic and Reconstructive Surgery, University of Florida College of Medicine, Gainesville, FL, USA

Ashley Titan Division of Plastic Surgery, Department of Surgery, Stanford University, Stanford, CA, USA

Sarah Townsley Mayo Clinic, Rochester, MN, USA

Eric R. Wagner Department of Orthopaedic Surgery, Emory University School of Medicine, Atlanta, GA, USA

Kitty Y. Wu Plastic and Hand Surgeon, Mayo Clinic, Rochester, MN, USA

Department of Orthopedic Surgery, Mayo Clinic, Rochester, MN, USA

Joanne Y. Zhou Department of Orthopaedic Surgery, Emory University School of Medicine, Atlanta, GA, USA

Chapter 1
Dupuytren's Contracture History and Considerations

Kier M. Blevins, Joanne Y. Zhou, and Eric R. Wagner

1.1 Origin and Historical Spread of Dupuytren's Disease

Dupuytren's disease is a fibrosing proliferative disorder of the hand palmar fascia often coined the "Viking disease" partly from its association and historical prevalence within Nordic regions and ethnic groups of Northern Europe [1, 2]. Owing its name to famed French surgeon, Baron Guillaume Dupuytren, Dupuytren's disease forms cords within the palm resulting in flexion contractures at the small joints of the hand which, although benign, can often become debilitating. The earliest references of the disease were from the eleventh century during the Age of the Vikings in Norsemen with bent fingers now thought to be descriptions of Dupuytren's Disease [3–5].

The origin and spread of Dupuytren's has been outlined by the movement of certain populations of interest by Robert McFarlane dating back to Indo-European migrations as early as 8000 BC where groups traveled from Asia Minor to Europe in search of areas able to sustain greater population growth [1]. These groups of interest as well as their historical interactions included the Celts, Germanic tribes, Romans, and later the Vikings.

The overall genetic make-up of central Europe was quite similar by 3000 BC and the great movements of groups continued with Celtic migration (1500 BC) from Anatolia and Germanic migration (1200 BC) into Europe and Northeast Europe from Caucasus [1, 6, 7]. The Roman empires conquest in Europe led to the defeat of the Celts in 50 BC where they fled to Cornwall, Wales, and Brittany [1, 8]. While occupying Europe and England for many years, the Romans never entered Scotland, Scandinavia, or Ireland which supports the lack of Dupuytren's descriptions in

K. M. Blevins · J. Y. Zhou · E. R. Wagner (✉)
Department of Orthopaedic Surgery, Emory University School of Medicine,
Atlanta, GA, USA
e-mail: eric.r.wagner@emory.edu

M. B. Gottschalk et al. (eds.), *Dupuytren's Disease*,
https://doi.org/10.1007/978-3-031-85873-4_1

Roman or Greek historical literature [1, 5, 9]. The Germanic tribes mixed with the Celts in war and then subsequently the Romans following the Celts defeat but there remains no archaeological evidence that the Romans genetically acquired and spread Dupuytren's disease through Northen Europe [1, 10].

Vikings were a group of Germanic tribes who were wayfarers and voyagers but never a formal migration of people. They mixed genetically among populations through raids and piracy and opportunistic movement along the northern coasts and great rivers through Europe. Many believe the Vikings caused the spread of Dupuytren's genes geographically during the eighth through thirteenth century [1]. It is important to understand both the movements and interactions of these groups temporally to gain insight on the development of genetic alterations and sporadic mutations giving rise to this complex, multifactorial disease.

1.2 Initial Description and Symbolism: Felix Platter, Curse of MacCrimmons, and the Hand of Benediction

The earliest published description of Dupuytren's disease was first by the Swiss physician Felix Platter who described characteristic palmar nodules and contractures in a stone mason in 1614 [11, 12]. His initial understanding was that inciting trauma raised flexor tendons from their sheaths inciting contractures forming the characteristic cords we know today. The British anatomist and physician Henry Cline almost 200 years later (coincidentally around the time of Guillaume Dupuytren's birth) showed these contractures and cords arose from the palmar fascia of the hand and not the flexor tendons themselves [12].

Around the same time of Platter's first observations in Switzerland during the seventeenth century, the MacCrimmons of the Western Isles of Scotland were thought to be cursed with a condition that bent the small finger significantly impairing their ability to play the bagpipes [11, 12]. This was known as the "Curse of the MacCrimmons" or "Cruimein Curse" in the 1650s, as the family were musicians to the chieftains of the clan Macleod of Skye [12]. There are many stories regarding the curse, including ones originating from a widow's son who was taken or others from a MacCrimmon woman Annag who was punished for giving secrets away to another clan. However, to date there are no known surviving members of the clan or factual evidence of the disease, other than these legends. Nonetheless, with a high prevalence of Dupuytren's disease in this population and the stories of bent fingers in this famous bagpiper clan, the curse has been correlated in history with the disease [12].

Dupuytren's contracture of the small and ring finger has also been debated regarding its presence in Christian symbolism [12, 13]. The Hand of Benediction may have been inspired by an earlier pope who suffered from Dupuytren's disease. However, Roman artifacts with similar hand positioning, such as the hand of Sabazios, predate the appearance of these symbols in Christianity, possibly arguing against this theory. Accordingly, instead of being the result of the disease, the Hand of Benediction portrayed with the partially flexed proximal joints of the ring and small fingers may have been a superimposition of Roman empire influence on the Christian church following its adoption of the religion in the fourth century [12]. Additionally, modern-day hand positioning and images of the pope do not reflect gestures similar to or imagery like the Hand of Benediction further adding to the mystery of its origin.

1.3 Key Players: Henry Cline, Astley Cooper, and Guillaume Dupuytren

Henry Cline's 1777 description and notes on Dupuytren's disease were uncovered and described by David Elliot, an English hand surgeon, in 1988 from the library of St. Thomas Hospital Medical School in London [12]. Earlier references in English, Irish, and Scandinavian literature may have existed, but no longer remain due to destruction of medical text and historic literature during the Viking raids of the ninth century. Additionally, the disease is most predominated in older populations and the decreased life expectancy of the times may have affected the disease prevalence.

Cline's notes from his dissection of two diseased cadaveric hands in 1777 were the first understanding linking the palmar fascia to the characteristic contractures [12]. He described the first fasciectomy as treatment in separating the fascia of the hand. However, his interpretation of the disease etiology may have been incorrect. He thought it originated due to traumatic sequelae and it was a disease primarily of laborers. He also was the first to describe treatment with sudden forceful extension (known as manipulation in modern times) of the fingers as documented in lecture notes from Thomas Smart in 1787 [12].

Sir Astley Cooper, a British surgeon and pupil of Cline, performed joint lectures of anatomy and surgery with Henry Cline at St. Thomas Hospital during the years of 1784–1811 [12]. During that time, notes available from visiting surgeons or students document only a few mentions, mostly asides, on contractures that may develop in the palmar fascia and a devised treatment for them. Additionally, Cooper wrote on contractures of the palmar aponeurosis of the hand and a subsequent dividing treatment of the bands in a small segment of a chapter in his book *A Treatise on Dislocations and Fractures of the Joints* in 1822 [12, 14].

Apart from Cooper and Cline's lectures, dissection notes and tangential mentions, there was no singular, formal medical publication with a narrowed focus on the palmar fascia contractures and treatment. It was not until Guillaume Dupuytren's lecture on December fifth in 1831 at Hôtel Dieu that any direct discussion was had on such topic of what we now know as Dupuytren's disease [15, 16]. He presented an ~40-year-old coachman, Jean-Joseph Demarteau, with almost 90-degree contractures of the small and ring finger joints of the hand. In his clinical lecture, he exclaims his discovery of the disease without any prior knowledge of it in medical literature and how it occurs without inciting trauma and its natural history. He performs releases of the fibrous bands in front of his audience and upon extension of the fingers a loud cracking sound arises for the finale of his demonstration.

Dupuytren shortly after published his findings in the Weekly Journal in Medicine and Surgery along with several others including an editorial in the English Journal The Lancet that sparked criticism of his newfound knowledge [15, 16]. The editor of The Lancet following Dupuytren's editorial in 1832 openly criticized Dupuytren for his unlikely lack of knowledge regarding teachings previously on the disease by his "brother in surgery", Astley Cooper [16, 17]. Both Dupuyten and Cooper knew each other professionally, and Dupuytren had visited Cooper in London at Guy's Hospital in 1826 accompanying him on rounds and through the wards [12]. Dupuytren's comment of only seeing 40 cases in 20 years that he treated without surgical intervention until 1831 may affirm his true lack of knowledge regarding the condition and treatment previously known to Cline and Cooper [18].

Dupuytren historically has been criticized for not giving credit to both Cline and Cooper's initial teachings. In a change of fate in history, we may have been writing on Cline's contracture or Cooper's Contracture, however there are important points to consider regarding the spread of knowledge during that era. London's medical press was much less endowed and organized by comparison to Parisian medical journals with weekly press. Elliot argues that Cline was from an entirely different generation [12]. His work was uncovered through third-party writings from his lectures and notes, not formal journal publications. This was a time before the advent of vibrant medical journalism that flourished in Paris by contrast to London during Cooper's era of ascendency into surgical prowess [12].

Eventually the years following Dupuytren's lecture and publications in 1832, vitriol controversy erupted regarding the origin of the disease description and pathophysiology with more opposition on the French front compared to English counterparts [16]. Glicenstein points out that the late recognition may have been due to the fact that "Dupuytren was feared, admired but hated by most of his French colleagues" [16].

It wasn't until the latter parts of the nineteenth century that many French surgeons' writings began to agree with Dupuytren on the palmar aponeurosis disease origin and his description [19–21]. And it wasn't until after his death that Nicaise gave mention to his name in 1874 and then Madelung in 1875. It was Ulysse Trelat's publication in 1887 that would finally give rise to the universally accepted eponym "Dupuytren's disease" [19–21]. The J. T. Hueston quote summarizes why Dupuytren's name is forever eponymous with the disease from that historic lecture in 1831: "Thoroughness of his demonstration, the brilliance of the presentation and the supremacy of his surgical authority combined to link permanently the name of Dupuytren with this hand deformity" [16, 22].

1.4 Epidemiology, Genetics, and Pathophysiology

The global reported prevalence for Dupuytren's contracture is 8.2% of the world's population with it being mostly predominant in men [23]. There is an increased association in individuals with excess alcohol use, diabetes, and metabolic syndromes, and the prevalence in alcoholic patients and those with diabetes has been shown to be as high as 24% and 34% respectively [24]. It is a multifactorial disease with no specific gene or allele implicated as seen in standard Mendelian inheritance models, although candidate genes involved are those in Wnt signaling, collagen, and extracellular matrix proteins [25]. Its inheritance pattern is autosomal dominant with variable penetrance and although commonly seen in descendants from Northern Europe, it has shown to be sporadic with a high prevalence in other geographic locations that are likely unrelated genetically [26–28].

Some examples of this are Dupuytren's disease having been identified in sub-Saharan African people of purely Afrodescent without genetic roots in Northern European populations of Scandinavia, Ireland, and England [28]. Egawa et al. also described a prevalence of 12% in Asian populations within Japan with uncertain genetic linkage to migrations from Europe [27]. The meta-analysis by Salari et al. showed the highest prevalence of the disease globally to be within Africa with a prevalence of 17.2% [23]. All of these demonstrate the increased environmental and epigenetic factors playing a substantial role in the development of the disease.

The pathophysiology of Dupuytren's is from aberrant architecture formation and fibrous tissue deposition by myofibroblastic cells [29]. There are three main stages of Dupuytren's contracture. First, the proliferative stage occurs forming a whorled pattern of immature myofibroblasts [25]. Second, the involution stage allows for tension-guided longitudinal formation of fibroblasts and then lastly, the residual stage leads to contracture deformity with acellular collagenous cord formation [25].

1.5 Conclusion

Dupuytren's contractures have a history full of famous legends and stories, rooted in the earliest medical textbooks and lectures. The genetics and pathophysiology are still poorly understood, as demonstrated by the mysterious roots in mythology and medical textbooks. This sets up the following chapters to help illustrate the many advances in our understanding of this pathologic process and novel treatments to improve the hand function of patients all over the world.

References

1. McFarlane RM. On the origin and spread of Dupuytren's disease. J Hand Surg Am. 2002;27(3):385–90.
2. Gil JA, Akelman MR, Hresko AM, Akelman E. Current concepts in the management of Dupuytren disease of the hand. J Am Acad Orthop Surg. 2021;29(11):462.
3. Hueston J. Dupuytren's contracture: medicolegal aspects. Med J Aust. 1987;147:S1–S11.
4. Jozsa LRA, Salamon A. A Dupuytren betegseg tortenete. Magyar Traumatol. 1997;1:11–4.
5. Flatt AE. The Vikings and Baron Dupuytren's disease. Proc (Bayl Univ Med Cent). 2001;14(4):378–84.
6. Early PF. Population studies in dupuytren's contracture. J Bone Joint Surg Br. 1962;44-B(3):602–13.
7. Hueston JT. Dupuytren's contracture – the trend to conser-vatism. Ann Roy Coll Surg Engl. 1965;36:134–51.
8. MacCullogh JA. The Celtic and Scandinavian religions. Westport: Greenwood; 1973. p. 9–12.
9. Paor D. The peoples of Ireland. London: Hutchinson; 1986.
10. Gummere FB. Germanic origins. A study in primitive culture. New York: C. Scribner's Sons; 1892.
11. Belusa L, Selzer AM, Partecke BD. Description of Dupuytren disease by the Basel physician and anatomist Felix Plater in 1614. Handchir Mikrochir Plast Chir. 1995;27(5):272–5.
12. Elliot D. The early history of contracture of the palmar fascia: part 1: the origin of the disease: the curse of the MacCrimmons: the hand of benediction: cline's contracture. J Hand Surg Br Eur. 1988;13(3):246–53.
13. Zdilla MJ. The hand of Sabazios: evidence of Dupuytren's disease in antiquity and the origin of the hand of benediction. J Hand Surg Asian Pac. 2017;22(3):403–10.
14. Burch D. Astley Paston Cooper (1768-1841): anatomist, radical and surgeon. J R Soc Med. 2010;103(12):505–8.
15. Welch CE. Guillaume Dupuytren: a surgeon in his place and time. JAMA. 1985;253(17):2584.
16. Glicenstein J. Dupuytren's disease – the story of an eponym. Chir Main. 2012;31(3):107–12.
17. Dupuytren. Retraction of the fingers producted by an affection of the palmar fascia. Lancet. 1834;2:222–5.
18. Thurston A. Dupuytren's disease or Cooper's contracture?: Kenneth Fitzpatrick Russell Memorial Lecture. ANZ J Surg. 2003;73(7):529–35.
19. Glicenstein J. Maladie de Dupuytren, histoire d'un éponyme. Chir Main. 2012;31(3):107–12.
20. Madelung O. An aetiologie and die operative Behandlung der Dupuytren'schen fingerverkrümmnung. Berl Klin Woch. 1875;12:191–3. [207–8]
21. Nicaise E. Étiologie de la contracture de Dupuytren. Bull Soc Anat Paris. 1874;43:379.
22. Hueston J. Dupuytren's contracture, vol. 31. Baltimore: Williams Wilkins; 1963. p. 66.
23. Salari N, Heydari M, Hassanabadi M, et al. The worldwide prevalence of the Dupuytren disease: a comprehensive systematic review and meta-analysis. J Orthop Surg Res. 2020;15(1):495.
24. Grazina R, Teixeira S, Ramos R, Sousa H, Ferreira A, Lemos R. Dupuytren's disease: where do we stand? EFORT Open Rev. 2019;4(2):63–9.
25. Aissvarya S, Ling KH, Arumugam M, Thilakavathy K. Molecular genetics of Dupuytren's contracture. EFORT Open Rev. 2024;9(8):723–32.
26. Michou L, Lermusiaux JL, Teyssedou JP, Bardin T, Beaudreuil J, Petit-Teixeira E. Genetics of Dupuytren's disease. Joint Bone Spine. 2012;79(1):7–12.
27. Egawa THH, Senrui H. Dupuytren's contracture in Japan. In: Hueston JT, Tubiana R, editors. Dupuyren's disease. Edinburgh: Churchill Livingstone; 1985.
28. Coulibaly NF, Doumbia MM, Dembele B, et al. Dupuytren's disease: a reality in Black Africa. Hand Surg Rehabil. 2020;39(5):448–53.
29. Walthall J, Anand P, Rehman UH. Dupuytren contracture. StatPearls; 2024.

Chapter 2
Pathophysiology and Genetic Considerations

Conner J. McMains and Alexander R. Graf

2.1 Cellular Pathophysiology

2.1.1 Myofibroblast Activity

The cellular pathophysiology of Dupuytren's disease (DD) centers around the pivotal role of myofibroblasts. These cells orchestrate a fibroproliferative response within the palmar fascia that creates pathologic nodules, cords, and joint contractures [1]. These cells, characterized by their expression of α-smooth muscle actin (α-SMA), play a role in collagen synthesis, extracellular matrix (ECM) composition, and intracellular mechanical interactions which shape the fibrotic changes observed in the disease [2]. Culture tests suggest the multiplying myofibroblasts in Dupuytren's tissue are derived from fibroblasts, and so behave partially as a normal fibroblast and partially as a transformed fibroblast [3, 4]. These cells lose expression of the epidermal growth factor receptor (EGFR), which suggests that they are not derived from the skin but from the connective tissue of the palmar fascia [2].

Dupuytren's disease typically progresses through three stages: proliferative, involutional, and residual [5]. Each of these stages is characterized by specific cellular events that result in different clinical manifestations (Fig. 2.1). During the proliferative stage, fibroblasts divide under the influence of fibroblast growth factor (FGF) from endothelial cells and as a result palmar nodules may be observed [6–8]. These cells contribute to excessive type I and type III collagen deposition and fibrosis, disrupting the balance between ECM synthesis and degradation. Moreover, in

---

C. J. McMains
Department of Plastic Surgery, Medical College of Wisconsin, Milwaukee, WI, USA

A. R. Graf (✉)
Department of Orthopedic Surgery, Hand and Upper Extremity Division, Medical College of Wisconsin, Milwaukee, WI, USA

M. B. Gottschalk et al. (eds.), *Dupuytren's Disease*,
https://doi.org/10.1007/978-3-031-85873-4_2

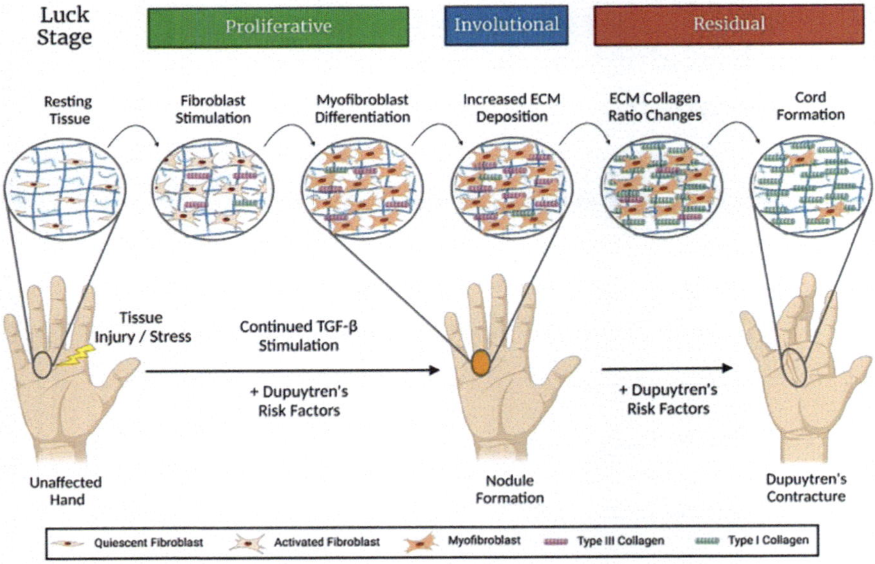

Fig. 2.1 Pathophysiology of Dupuytren's contracture. DD progression exists on histologic, cellular, and clinical levels. Resting tissue of the unaffected hand contains quiescent fibroblasts. Upon tissue injury or stress, fibroblasts are activated, proliferate, and differentiate into mature myofibroblasts (proliferative stage). With continued TGF-β stimulation and DD risk factors, disease progresses. Nodule formation occurs as myofibroblasts differentiate and produce extracellular matrix (ECM), with collagen III:I ratio predominating (Involutional stage). The ECM collagen ratio changes to I:III, increased collagen crosslinking occurs, and cellularity decreases as cords form and contraction ensues (residual stage). TGF, transforming growth factor. (Used with permission from [9].

the proliferative stage, type III collagen predominates over type I [6]. Later, during the involutional phase, myofibroblasts originate from the transformation of quiescent fibroblasts via a process known as fibroblast to myofibroblast transition [1]. This transformation is driven by complex signaling networks, prominently featuring the cytokine TGF-β [10]. Local ischemia and oxygen radicals may also influence the fibroblast to myofibroblast cell transformation [11]. Upon activation, myofibroblasts exhibit heightened contractile activity which can act on the extracellular matrix (ECM), fostering the formation of fibrous cords that tether the palmar fascia to the dermis and tendons. This contractile force leads to the characteristic digital contractures seen in DD (Fig. 2.1).

In the residual phase, the cords become hypocellular and more closely resemble scar tissue. Nodules may regress during this stage [12]. Myofibroblasts, through cytokine signaling, influence the expression and activity of matrix metalloproteinases (MMPs) and their inhibitors, tissue inhibitors of metalloproteinases (TIMPs) [13]. ECM remodeling involves a balance between MMPs and TIMPs. Dysregulation in the MMPs/TIMPs ratio tips the scale toward excessive ECM accumulation. This imbalance results in a net increase in collagen deposition, reinforcing the fibrotic changes.

ADAMs (A disintegrin and metalloproteinase) and ADAMTS (A disintegrin and metalloproteinase with thrombospondin motifs) are groups of zinc-dependent metalloproteinases that are involved in several tissue pathologies including inflammatory disorders, lung and cardiovascular disease, and cancer metastasis. They regulate cell proliferation, migration, apoptosis, and extracellular matrix remodeling [14]. An imbalance among these proteins has been implicated in the fibrosis and contracture that occur in DD [15]. In one series of 12 patients with inoperable gastric carcinoma treated with Marimastat, a synthetic MMP inhibitor, half developed adhesive capsulitis of the shoulder or Dupuytren disease [16]. Levels of gene expression of several MMPs and ADAMTS proteins have been correlated with recurrence of fixed flexion deformity after fasciectomy at 14-month follow-up [17]. Townley et al. showed that the MMP inhibitor ilomostat reduced fibroblast-mediated contraction in Dupuytren's nodule and cord tissue samples [18]. MMPs may represent a useful target to prevent recurring contracture in DD.

Myofibroblasts also express integrin receptors that bind to fibronectin (an ECM protein), mediating cell-cell attachment and signaling [19]. In Dupuytren's contractures, myofibroblasts contribute to the deposition of fibronectin, altering the composition of the ECM [20]. An in vitro study revealed that diseased cells respond more dramatically to isometric tension by altering levels of β-catenin and fibronectin in the ECM [21]. Additionally, α5β1 integrin has been detected in highly cellular tissue within the proliferative and involutional phases [22]. This integrin is downregulated in hypocellular tissue in the involutional and residual phases. Alteration in fibronectin-integrin expression influences cell adhesion, migration, and matrix remodeling, ultimately contributing to progression of the contractile processes in DD [23]. Connective tissue growth factor (CTGF), a downstream mediator of TGF-β, amplifies fibrotic responses by stimulating collagen synthesis and ECM deposition [24].

2.1.2 *Cell Signaling*

The development and progression of DD requires a dynamic interplay between multiple cell signaling pathways. Together, these cytokines and chemokines orchestrate fibrotic responses within the affected tissues. As discussed, TGF-β plays a prominent role in fibroblast activation, myofibroblast differentiation, and stimulation of extracellular matrix synthesis through the β-catenin pathway [25]. Its downstream effects include increased collagen production and decreased collagen degradation, culminating in the characteristic fibrous cords of DD [26].

Interleukin-6 (IL-6) is another important mediator that plays a key role in inflammation and tissue remodeling. IL-6 promotes fibroblast proliferation and myofibroblast differentiation, perpetuating fibrosis through enhanced ECM synthesis [27]. Moreover, IL-6 contributes to the recruitment of immune cells, sustaining the inflammatory milieu that fuels the disease process [28]. Tumor necrosis factor-alpha (TNF-α), a potent pro-inflammatory cytokine, amplifies the fibrotic cascade in Dupuytren's Disease. TNF-α contributes to fibroblast activation and myofibroblast differentiation, while also enhancing the production of MMPs that mediate ECM degradation [28, 29]. Dysregulated balance between MMPs and their inhibitors further tips the scale toward fibrosis [13]. Chemokines, such as C-C motif chemokine ligand 11 (CCL11) play a role in recruiting immune cells and promoting inflammation within the diseased tissue [30]. Sphingosine-1-phosphate, a signaling sphingolipid, has been shown to promote fibroblast activity in Dupuytren's disease by the activation of the S1P2 receptor, activating NMMII (non-muscle myosin II) present in high concentrations in Dupuytren's nodules [31].

Emerging evidence highlights the influence of hormones on Dupuytren's disease pathogenesis. Dupuytren's cords have been found to express androgen receptors, which may explain the disease's male predominance. In an in vitro study by Pagnotta et al. androgen receptors were more often detected by immunostaining in cell nuclei of DD myofibroblasts than in normal palmar fascia fibroblasts. In addition, androgen receptors co-localized with alpha-actin in both cell cultures and tissue samples [32]. On the other hand, estrogen and progesterone receptors have not been found in palmar fascia tissue samples [33]. Nonetheless, tamoxifen, a selective estrogen receptor modulator and inhibitor of TGF-β activity, downregulates TGF-β2 protein in cultured diseased cord fibroblasts and decreases their contractile function [34]. Palmar fascia tissue from patients with DD cultured with 5-alpha dihydrotestosterone (5α-DHT) showed greater fibroblast proliferation and strong expression of anti-α-smooth muscle actin [35]. Androgens may induce myofibroblast differentiation and proliferation as well as modulate palmar fascial growth and development [32]. Insulin-like growth factor-2 (IGF-2), a hormone with structural similarity to insulin, also regulates cellular contractility in Dupuytren's disease [36]. IGF-2 has been shown in cell culture to enhance fibroblast contractility in DD cells [37]. While TGF-β1 and IGF-2 have combinatorial effects on myofibroblast differentiation in murine models, this was not present in human cells. IGF binding protein-6 (IGFBP-6) mRNA and protein levels are attenuated in Dupuytren's disease cells and tissue. IGFBP-6 has been shown to inhibit DD cell proliferation [37].

2.2 Genetic Underpinnings

Dupuytren's disease is most often inherited in an autosomal dominant pattern with variable penetrance; however, rare X-linked, mitochondrial, and recessive inheritance patterns have also been described [25, 38, 39].

Genetic investigations into DD have illuminated a spectrum of genes implicated in its pathogenesis. Previous genome-wide association studies (GWAS) have shown a genetic association of DD with chromosomes 6, 11, and 16 [25, 40]. Additional genomic variations in patients with DD have been reported, including associations with the HLA-DRB1*15 allele and a mutation in the rRNA 16 s in a cohort of patients with mitochondrial inheritance [25]. Recently, the largest GWAS in DD to date revealed 26 predisposing variants [41].

The Wnt family of genes encodes for glycoproteins that engage in extracellular signaling [42]. Wnts activate β-catenin in the cell nucleus, which change gene expression that influences cell proliferation [43]. While β-catenin is upregulated in DD, it is not mutated [44]. Dolmans et al. identified nine chromosomal loci associated with DD in their GWAS. These included Wnt signaling pathway genes WNT2, WNT4, SFRP4, SULF1, WNT7B, and RSPO2 [45]. Another study by Mosakhani et al. noted numerous microRNAs that restrain the β-catenin pathway, WNT5A, ZIC1, and TGFB1 [46].

The COL5A1 gene encodes collagen type V alpha-1 chain, an essential component of the ECM [47]. After immature collagen is processed by extracellular enzymes to create mature collagen fibrils, type V collagen regulates the width of these fibrils [48]. Mutations in the COL5A1 gene cause Ehlers-Danlos syndrome, whereas COL5A1 expression is increased in DD nodule tissue [49]. Increased expression of COL1A1, COL1A2, COL5A1, and COL6A1 has been found in nodule tissue compared to cord tissue. Cord tissue also contains higher levels of collagen cross-linking [49].

A DNA microarray analysis by Chang et al. found upregulation of MafB (musculoaponeurotic fibrosarcoma oncogene homolog B), collagen type V, α-2 (COL5A2), collagen type VIII, α-1 (COL8A1), contactin I (CNTN1), and leucine-rich repeat containing 17 (LRRC17) in DD cord tissue compared to normal tissue from healthy patients with carpal tunnel syndrome [50]. Diseased tissue had a fourfold increase in MafB which was localized in cells which also expressed α-smooth muscle actin. MafB is a protein encoded by the Maf oncogene which influences cellular differentiation and tissue development and can be influenced by Hox proteins [51]. Dupuytren's disease is similar histologically to fibrosarcoma in its early stages, adding validity to the role of the MafB gene in disease development [52].

The TGFBR2 gene encodes the TGF-β receptor type II, a central regulator of fibrosis [53]. Dysfunctional TGF-β signaling, often stemming from genetic variations, leads to an imbalance between ECM synthesis and degradation, fostering excessive collagen accumulation. This shared pathway contributes to fibrosis in both DD and related conditions, highlighting the centrality of TGF-β signaling in fibrotic disorders [53]. Recently, verteporfin has been used in vitro to halt differentiation of fibroblasts into myofibroblasts in nodules from Dupuytren's patients through inhibition of TGF-β-mediated signaling [54]. However, no clinical studies have been performed to date. Exogenous TGF-β2 added to a Dupuytren's disease cord has been shown in vitro to increase collagen, DNA, and protein production. This effect was blocked by TGF-β2 neutralizing antibody [34]. Through the use of an ELISA assay, a 2.5-fold increase in TGF-β2 protein in Dupuytren's disease cords was found compared to normal fascia obtained during carpal tunnel release surgery [55]. Case–control studies have explored the possible association between DD susceptibility and single nucleotide polymorphisms (TNPs) in the transforming growth factor TGF-β pathway, but no SNPs were found to influence TGF-β1, TGF-β2 and, TGF-β receptors I-III [56].

Table 2.1 Molecular abnormalities in Dupuytren's disease

Molecular abnormality	Change
Cytokines and growth factors	
TGF-β [46, 86]	↑
IL- [86]	↑
bFGF [8, 86]	↑
PDGF [22, 87]	↑
ECM-associated proteins	
Collagen [88]	↑
β-catenin [38]	↑
α5β1 integrin [18]	↑
Fibronectin [17, 38]	↑
MMPs and associated proteins	
MMP -2, -14 [35, 41, 50–52]	↑
TIMP-1, -2 [13, 50]	↑
MMP-3, -27 [14, 89]	↓
TIMP-2, -3, -4 [14]	↓
ADAMTS-1, -6, 18, -19, -20 [14]	↓

Beyond these central genes, numerous other loci have been implicated through further genome-wide association. These include genes involved in ECM regulation (e.g., ITGA11, LOXL4, EPDR1), cell adhesion (e.g., VCAM1, CADM1, CHI3L1, THBS4), and extracellular matrix remodeling (MMP2, MMP14) [41, 47, 57–59]. Collectively, these genes underpin the complexity of DD pathogenesis, reflecting a coordinated interplay of molecular players involved in fibroproliferation and ECM dysregulation (Table 2.1).

2.3 Associated Co-morbidities

DD has been associated with several conditions, including diabetes mellitus, epilepsy, tobacco use, AIDS, liver disease, low body mass index, adhesive capsulitis, and vascular disorders [60–62]. It also shares a close relationship with nonmelanoma skin cancer, psoriasis, and has been associated with increased risk of cancer and overall mortality [63, 64].

The insulin resistance and hyperglycemia in diabetes mellitus (DM) create chronic systemic inflammation and microvascular injury which are conducive to tissue fibrosis and nodules and cord development in DD [65]. The pathophysiologic process is similar to that found in diabetic neuropathy, retinopathy, and nephropathy [66]. In the general adult population, there is approximately a 2–6% prevalence of DD while in patients with diabetes, the prevalence is as high as 10–15% [67, 68]. Patients with type 1 diabetes may be at higher risk, but this association has not been proven [69]. Hyperglycemia promotes formation of advanced glycated end products (AGEs), which are also associated with fibroproliferative disorders and other complications from DM [70]. Higher levels of AGEs in DD palmar fascia increase collagen deposition and collagen stiffness [71]. DM also increases the formation of myofibroblasts [72].

DD has been associated with epilepsy both due to chronic exposure to anticonvulsant medication as well as heritable genes [73, 74]. Chronic administration of the anticonvulsant medication phenobarbital has been shown to simulate tissue growth factors and postulated to influence DD development after 20 years of medication usage [75, 76]. The association between epilepsy and Dupuytren disease has been observed since 1963 by Ling [77]. Early studies published were observational in nature, surveying patients in inpatient treatment wards, and the cause of the association is not clearly defined [78].

Currently, several acquired diseases or environmental factors may increase free radical deposition thus increasing the propensity for DD. Acquired immunodeficiency syndrome (AIDS), characterized by immune dysfunction, disrupts the body's surveillance mechanisms, promoting accumulation of free radicals and ECM remodeling [79]. Vascular disorders and smoking, through hypoxia and inflammation, escalate fibroblast activation and collagen synthesis in both DD and vascular pathologies [79]. This shared predisposition highlights the significance of microenvironmental factors in driving fibrosis.

2.4 Ethnology

DD displays a multifaceted ethnological distribution that has long intrigued researchers and clinicians alike. This condition predominantly affects individuals of Northern European descent, with an emphasis on populations from Scandinavian countries. In Denmark, up to 12% of the population over the age of 55 can be afflicted. Similar epidemiological patterns have been identified in other Northern European countries, such as Sweden, Norway, and the UK [80].

Throughout history, DD has been called the curse of the MacCrimmons in sixteenth-century Scotland as well as "Vikings disease" [81]. However, more recent GWAS have challenged the genetic evidence for a Viking origin of Dupuytren's disease [82]. However, incidence of DD is exceedingly rare in many Asian countries and among black individuals [83]. This global prevalence underscores the interplay between genetic predisposition and environmental factors.

2.5 Environmental Factors Influence Pathophysiology

Environmental factors intricately shape the cellular pathophysiology of DD, modulating the behavior of key cell types and contributing to the fibroproliferative process (Fig. 2.2). Nongenetic factors associated with DD include advanced age, male sex, family history, diabetes mellitus, heavy alcohol consumption, and manual work

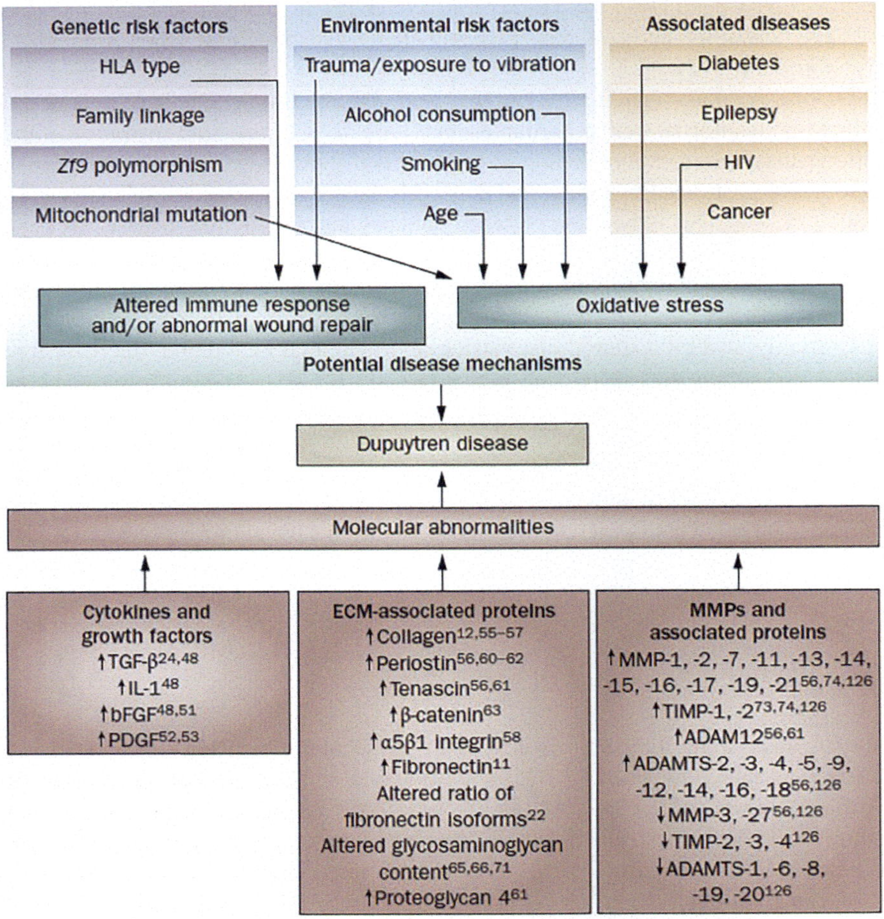

Fig. 2.2 Risk factors for Dupuytren's disease. (Used with permission from Shih et al. [56])

exposure in a dose-dependent manner [84]. Emerging evidence suggests that exposure to mechanical stress and trauma, particularly in individuals with a genetic predisposition, may increase the propensity for disease formation [85]. Repetitive microtrauma to the palmar fascia such as from vibration can lead to chronic tissue inflammation and activation of fibroblasts [86]. Under these conditions, fibroblasts receive cues from the altered extracellular matrix composition and the presence of pro-inflammatory cytokines, including TGF-β,TNF, IL-6, and IL-8 [28]. The exposure to TGF-β and other profibrotic factors triggers fibroblast activation and their transition into myofibroblasts. Myofibroblasts, in turn, generate excessive collagen and other extracellular matrix components, causing tissue stiffening and contraction. Currently, an intranodular injection of an anti-TNF antibody (adalimumab) is currently undergoing clinical trials for use in early-stage DD [29]. This is based on in vitro studies supporting adalimumab downregulating myofibroblast activity in a dose-dependent manner [28].

Vascular disorders and smoking, common coexisting conditions with DD, contribute to local tissue hypoxia and the increase of free radicals [56, 87]. Hypoxia-inducible factors (HIFs) play a critical role in orchestrating the cellular response to low oxygen levels [88]. Under hypoxic conditions, fibroblasts exhibit increased collagen synthesis, myofibroblast differentiation, and release of pro-fibrotic factors, ultimately exacerbating the fibrotic process [89]. However, a preliminary study demonstrated that the contractility of Dupuytren's fibroblasts was not influenced by treatment with elevated oxygen levels [90]. Nonetheless, aberrant angiogenesis and local tissue hypoxia may play a role in the pathophysiology of DD [89].

Viil et al. shed light on the significance of laminin-rich blood vessels as proliferation centers within the affected tissue. The study demonstrated that these specialized blood vessels display enhanced growth factor signaling, particularly involving factors such as TGF-β and platelet-derived growth factor (PDGF) [7]. The blood vessels not only provide a niche for fibroblast activation but also facilitate the recruitment of immune cells and inflammatory mediators, further perpetuating the microenvironment conducive to fibrosis. Microvascular damage has also been postulated as predisposing individuals to DD through exposure to an autoantigen, resulting in a T-cell-mediated autoimmune disorder [91]. This is supported by previous studies that have found dense T-cell infiltrates in DD nodules [91, 92]. Future studies aimed toward understanding these molecular mechanisms will afford more targeted interventions to disrupt this complex fibrotic cascade and curtail disease progression.

2.6 Treatment Implications: Fat Grafting and Adipose-Derived Stem Cells

The intricate interplay between cellular pathways and environmental factors opens avenues for innovative treatment strategies in DD. One promising approach involves the utilization of adipose-derived stem cells (ASCs) and fat grafting. A study by Verhoekx et al. sheds light on the potential of ASCs in inhibiting contractile myofibroblasts, thereby offering a novel therapeutic perspective [28]. ASCs, mesenchymal stem cells sourced from adipose tissue, exhibit remarkable regenerative and immunomodulatory properties [93]. These cells have the capacity to differentiate into various cell lineages, including fibroblasts, myofibroblasts, and adipocytes. The study by Verhoekx et al. revealed that ASCs exert an inhibitory effect on the contractile activity of myofibroblasts. This effect was attributed to the paracrine secretion of factors, such as hepatocyte growth factor (HGF) and IL-10, which suppress TGF-β-driven myofibroblast activation [94].

The use of fat grafting not only provides a scaffold for ASCs but also delivers growth factors and cytokines present in adipose tissue. When ASCs in platelet-rich plasma (PRP) are co-cultured with Dupuytren myofibroblasts, markers of fibrosis and the contractile cell phenotype are reduced [95]. These factors contribute to local tissue remodeling, ECM modulation, and immune modulation. By harnessing the regenerative potential of ASCs and the microenvironmental cues of adipose tissue, fat grafting holds promise as a therapeutic strategy that addresses both the cellular and environmental aspects of DD. However, future studies are warranted to validate its clinical efficacy before translation into widespread clinical use.

2.7 Conclusion

The associations between DD and coexisting conditions reveal a network of shared pathways and common molecular mechanisms that transcend disease boundaries. This interplay underscores the significance of genetic predisposition and environmental influences in shaping disease presentation and progression. By examining these parallels, researchers may unravel novel therapeutic avenues that target overarching molecular pathways, offering hope for interventions that address not only DD but also its related conditions.

References

1. Gabbiani G, Majno G. Dupuytren's contracture: fibroblast contraction? An ultrastructural study. Am J Pathol. 1972;66:131–46.
2. Tomasek JJ, Schultz RJ, Episalla CW, Newman SA. The cytoskeleton and extracellular matrix of the Dupuytren's disease "myofibroblast": an immunofluorescence study of a nonmuscle cell type. J Hand Surg Am. 1986;11:365–71. https://doi.org/10.1016/S0363-5023(86)80143-5.
3. Skalli O, Schürch W, Seemayer T, Lagacé R, Montandon D, Pittet B, Gabbiani G. Myofibroblasts from diverse pathologic settings are heterogeneous in their content of actin isoforms and intermediate filament proteins. Lab Investig. 1989;60:275–85.
4. Moyer KE, Banducci DR, Graham WP 3rd, Ehrlich HP. Dupuytren's disease: physiologic changes in nodule and cord fibroblasts through aging in vitro. Plast Reconstr Surg. 2002;110:187–6.
5. Luck JV. Dupuytren's contracture; a new concept of the pathogenesis correlated with surgical management. J Bone Joint Surg Am. 1959;41-A:635–64.
6. Alioto RJ, Rosier RN, Burton RI, Edward Puzas J. Comparative effects of growth factors on fibroblasts of Dupuytren's tissue and normal palmar fascia. J Hand Surg Am. 1994;19:442–52. https://doi.org/10.1016/0363-5023(94)90059-0.
7. Viil J, Maasalu K, Maemets-Allas K, Tamming L, Lohmussaar K, Tooming M, Ingerpuu S, Martson A, Jaks V. Laminin-rich blood vessels display activated growth factor signaling and act as the proliferation centers in Dupuytren's contracture. Arthritis Res Ther. 2015;17:144. https://doi.org/10.1186/s13075-015-0661-y.
8. Gonzalez AM, Buscaglia M, Fox R, Isacchi A, Sarmientos P, Farris J, Ong M, Martineau D, Lappi DA, Baird A. Basic fibroblast growth factor in Dupuytren's contracture. Am J Pathol. 1992;141:661–71.

9. Lambi AG, Morrell NT, Popoff SN, Benhaim P, Barbe MF. Let's Focus on the Fibrosis in Dupuytren Disease: Cell Communication Network Factor 2 as a Novel Target. J Hand Surg Glob Online. 2023;5(5):682–688. https://doi.org/10.1016/j.jhsg.2023.06.017.
10. Kloen P, Jennings CL, Gebhardt MC, Springfield DS, Mankin HJ. Transforming growth factor-β: Possible roles in Dupuytren's contracture. J Hand Surg Am. 1995;20:101–8. https://doi.org/10.1016/S0363-5023(05)80067-X.
11. Murrell G, Francis M, Howlett C. Dupuytren's contracture. Fine structure in relation to aetiology. J Bone Joint Surg Br. 1989;71-B:367–73. https://doi.org/10.1302/0301-620X.71B3.2722922.
12. Grazina R, Teixeira S, Ramos R, Sousa H, Ferreira A, Lemos R. Dupuytren's disease: where do we stand? EFORT Open Rev. 2019;4:63–9. https://doi.org/10.1302/2058-5241.4.180021.
13. Ratajczak-Wielgomas K, Gosk J, Rabczyński J, Augoff K, Podhorska-Okołów M, Gamian A, Rutowski R. Expression of MMP-2, TIMP-2, TGF-β1, and Decorin in Dupuytren's Contracture. Connect Tissue Res. 2012;53:469–77. https://doi.org/10.3109/03008207.2012.686542.
14. Wang Z, Li W, Chen S, Tang XX. Role of ADAM and ADAMTS proteases in pathological tissue remodeling. Cell Death Discov. 2023;9:447. https://doi.org/10.1038/s41420-023-01744-z.
15. Johnston P, Chojnowski AJ, Davidson RK, Riley GP, Donell ST, Clark IM. A complete expression profile of matrix-degrading metalloproteinases in Dupuytren's disease. J Hand Surg. 2007;32:343–51.
16. Hutchinson JW, Tierney GM, Parsons SL, Davis TRC. Dupuytren's disease and frozen shoulder induced by treatment with a matrix metalloproteinase inhibitor. Journal Bone Joint Surg Br. 1998;80-B:907–8. https://doi.org/10.1302/0301-620X.80B5.0800907.
17. Johnston P, Larson D, Clark IM, Chojnowski AJ. Metalloproteinase gene expression correlates with clinical outcome in Dupuytren's disease. J Hand Surg Am. 2008;33:1160–7. https://doi.org/10.1016/j.jhsa.2008.04.002.
18. Townley WA, Cambrey AD, Khaw PT, Grobbelaar AO. Matrix metalloproteinase inhibition reduces contraction by Dupuytren fibroblasts. J Hand Surg Am. 2008;33:1608–16. https://doi.org/10.1016/j.jhsa.2008.06.013.
19. Tomasek JJ, Schultz RJ, Haaksma CJ. Extracellular matrix-cytoskeletal connections at the surface of the specialized contractile fibroblast (myofibroblast) in Dupuytren disease. J Bone Joint Surg Am. 1987;69:1400–7.
20. Berndt A, Kosmehl H, Katenkamp D, Tauchmann V. Appearance of the myofibroblastic phenotype in Dupuytren's disease is associated with a fibronectin, laminin, collagen type IV and tenascin extracellular matrix. Pathobiology. 1994;62:55–8. https://doi.org/10.1159/000163879.
21. Howard JC, Varallo VM, Ross DC, Roth JH, Faber KJ, Alman B, Gan BS. Elevated levels of β-catenin and fibronectin in three-dimensional collagen cultures of Dupuytren's disease cells are regulated by tension in vitro. BMC Musculoskelet Disord. 2003;4:16. https://doi.org/10.1186/1471-2474-4-16.
22. Magro G, Lanzafame S, Micali G. Co-ordinate expression of alpha5 beta1 integrin and fibronectin in Dupuytren's disease. Acta Histochem. 1995;97:229–33. https://doi.org/10.1016/S0065-1281(11)80184-4.
23. Magro G, Fraggetta F, Travali S, Lanzafame S. Immunohistochemical expression and distribution of alpha2beta1, alpha6beta1, alpha5beta1 integrins and their extracellular ligands, type IV collagen, laminin and fibronectin in palmar fibromatosis. Gen Diagn Pathol. 1997;143:203–8.
24. Tripoli M, Cordova A, Moschella F. Update on the role of molecular factors and fibroblasts in the pathogenesis of Dupuytren's disease. J Cell Commun Signal. 2016;10:315–30. https://doi.org/10.1007/s12079-016-0331-0.
25. Michou L, Lermusiaux J-L, Teyssedou J-P, Bardin T, Beaudreuil J, Petit-Teixeira E. Genetics of Dupuytren's disease. Joint Bone Spine. 2012;79:7–12. https://doi.org/10.1016/j.jbspin.2011.05.027.
26. Badalamente MA, Sampson SP, Hurst LC, Dowd A, Miyasaka K. The role of transforming growth factor beta in Dupuytren's disease. J Hand Surg Am. 1996;21:210–5. https://doi.org/10.1016/S0363-5023(96)80102-X.

27. Johnson BZ, Stevenson AW, Prêle CM, Fear MW, Wood FM. The role of IL-6 in skin fibrosis and cutaneous wound healing. Biomedicines. 2020;8:101. https://doi.org/10.3390/biomedicines8050101.
28. Verjee LS, Verhoekx JSN, Chan JKK, Krausgruber T, Nicolaidou V, Izadi D, Davidson D, Feldmann M, Midwood KS, Nanchahal J. Unraveling the signaling pathways promoting fibrosis in Dupuytren's disease reveals TNF as a therapeutic target. Proc Natl Acad Sci USA. 2013;110:E928–37. https://doi.org/10.1073/pnas.1301100110.
29. Nanchahal J, Ball C, Davidson D, Williams L, Sones W, McCann FE, Cabrita M, Swettenham J, Cahoon NJ, Copsey B, Anne Francis E, Taylor PC, Black J, Barber VS, Dutton S, Feldmann M, Lamb SE. Anti-tumour necrosis factor therapy for dupuytren's disease: a randomised dose response proof of concept phase 2a clinical trial. EBioMedicine. 2018;33:282–8. https://doi.org/10.1016/j.ebiom.2018.06.022.
30. Bujak M, Ratkaj I, Markova-Car E, Jurišić D, Horvatić A, Vučinić S, Lerga J, Baus-Lončar M, Pavelić K, Kraljević Pavelić S. Inflammatory gene expression upon TGF-β1-induced p38 activation in primary Dupuytren's disease fibroblasts. Front Mol Biosci. 2015;2:68. https://doi.org/10.3389/fmolb.2015.00068.
31. Komatsu I, Bond J, Selim A, Tomasek JJ, Levin LS, Levinson H. dupuytren's fibroblast contractility by sphingosine-1-phosphate is mediated through non-muscle myosin II. J Hand Surg Am. 2010;35:1580–8. https://doi.org/10.1016/j.jhsa.2010.07.009.
32. Pagnotta A, Specchia N, Greco F. Androgen receptors in Dupuytren's contracture. J Orthop Res. 2002;20:163–8. https://doi.org/10.1016/S0736-0266(01)00072-9.
33. Hankin F, Eckenrode J, Louis D. Oestrogen and progesterone hormone receptors in Dupuytren's disease. J Hand Surg Am. 1986;11:463–4. https://doi.org/10.1016/0266-7681(86)90184-1.
34. Kuhn MA, Payne WG, Kierney PC, Pu LL, Smith PD, Siegler K, Ko F, Wang X, Robson MC. Cytokine manipulation of explanted Dupuytren's affected human palmar fascia. Int J Surg Investig. 2001;2:443–56.
35. Pagnotta A, Specchia N, Soccetti A, Manzotti S, Greco F. Responsiveness of Dupuytren's disease fibroblasts to 5 alpha-dihydrotestosterone. J Hand Surg Am. 2003;28:1029–34.
36. Raykha C, Crawford J, Gan BS, Fu P, Bach LA, O'Gorman DB. IGF-II and IGFBP-6 regulate cellular contractility and proliferation in Dupuytren's disease. Biochim Biophys Acta. 2013;1832:1511–9. https://doi.org/10.1016/j.bbadis.2013.04.018.
37. Raykha C, Crawford J, Gan BS, Fu P, Bach LA, O'Gorman DB. IGF-II and IGFBP-6 regulate cellular contractility and proliferation in Dupuytren's disease. Biochim Biophys Acta (BBA) Mol Basis Dis. 2013;1832:1511–9. https://doi.org/10.1016/j.bbadis.2013.04.018.
38. Bayat A, Walter J, Lambe H, Watson JS, Stanley JK, Marino M, Ferguson MWJ, Ollier WER. Identification of a novel mitochondrial mutation in Dupuytren's disease using multiplex DHPLC. Plast Reconstr Surg. 2005;115:134–41.
39. DiBenedetti DB, Nguyen D, Zografos L, Ziemiecki R, Zhou X. Prevalence, incidence, and treatments of Dupuytren's disease in the United States: results from a population-based study. Hand. 2011;6:149–58. https://doi.org/10.1007/s11552-010-9306-4.
40. Ojwang JO, Adrianto I, Gray-McGuire C, Nath SK, Sun C, Kaufman KM, Harley JB, Rayan GM. Genome-wide association scan of Dupuytren's disease. J Hand Surg Am. 2010;35:2039–45. https://doi.org/10.1016/j.jhsa.2010.08.008.
41. Ng M, Thakkar D, Southam L, Werker P, Ophoff R, Becker K, Nothnagel M, Franke A, Nurnberg P, Espirito-Santo AI, Izadi D, Hennies HC, Nanchahal J, Zeggini E, Furniss D. A genome-wide association study of Dupuytren disease reveals 17 additional variants implicated in fibrosis. Am J Hum Genet. 2017;101:417–27. https://doi.org/10.1016/j.ajhg.2017.08.006.
42. Zhang AY, Kargel JS. The basic science of Dupuytren disease. Hand Clin. 2018;34:301–5. https://doi.org/10.1016/j.hcl.2018.03.001.
43. Moon RT, Kohn AD, De Ferrari GV, Kaykas A. WNT and beta-catenin signalling: diseases and therapies. Nat Rev Genet. 2004;5:691–701. https://doi.org/10.1038/nrg1427.
44. Varallo VM, Gan BS, Seney S, Ross DC, Roth JH, Richards RS, McFarlane RM, Alman B, Howard JC. Beta-catenin expression in Dupuytren's disease: potential role for cell-matrix

interactions in modulating beta-catenin levels in vivo and in vitro. Oncogene. 2003;22:3680–4. https://doi.org/10.1038/sj.onc.1206415.
45. Dolmans GH, Werker PM, Hennies HC, Furniss D, Festen EA, Franke L, Becker K, van der Vlies P, Wolffenbuttel BH, Tinschert S, Toliat MR, Nothnagel M, Franke A, Klopp N, Wichmann H-E, Nürnberg P, Giele H, Ophoff RA, Wijmenga C. Wnt signaling and Dupuytren's disease. N Engl J Med. 2011;365:307–17. https://doi.org/10.1056/NEJMoa1101029.
46. Mosakhani N, Guled M, Lahti L, Borze I, Forsman M, Pääkkönen V, Ryhänen J, Knuutila S. Unique microRNA profile in Dupuytren's contracture supports deregulation of β-catenin pathway. Mod Pathol. 2010;23:1544–52. https://doi.org/10.1038/modpathol.2010.146.
47. Forrester HB, Temple-Smith P, Ham S, De Kretser D, Southwick G, Sprung CN. Genome-wide analysis using exon arrays demonstrates an important role for expression of extra-cellular matrix, fibrotic control and tissue remodelling genes in dupuytren's disease. PLoS One. 2013;8:e59056. https://doi.org/10.1371/journal.pone.0059056.
48. National Library of Medicine (US) (2017) COL5A1 gene. In: MedLine Plus. https://medlineplus.gov/genetics/gene/col5a1/. Accessed 11 Feb 2024
49. van Beuge MM, Ten Dam E-JPM, Werker PMN, et al. Matrix and cell phenotype differences in Dupuytren's disease. Fibrogenesis Tissue Repair. 2016;9:9. https://doi.org/10.1186/s13069-016-0046-0.
50. Lee LC, Zhang AY, Chong AK, Pham H, Longaker MT, Chang J. Expression of a novel gene, MafB, in Dupuytren's disease. J Hand Surg Am. 2006;31:211–8.
51. Kataoka K, Yoshitomo-Nakagawa K, Shioda S, Nishizawa M. A set of Hox proteins interact with the Maf oncoprotein to inhibit its DNA binding, transactivation, and transforming activities. J Biol Chem. 2001;276:819–26. https://doi.org/10.1074/jbc.M007643200.
52. Erdmann MW, Quaba AA, Sommerlad BC. Epithelioid sarcoma masquerading as Dupuytren's disease. Br J Plast Surg. 1995;48:39–42. https://doi.org/10.1016/0007-1226(95)90029-2.
53. Zhang AY, Fong KD, Pham H, Nacamuli RP, Longaker MT, Chang J. Gene expression analysis of Dupuytren's disease: the role of TGF-beta2. J Hand Surg Eur. 2008;33:783–90. https://doi.org/10.1177/1753193408091352.
54. Puerta Cavanzo N, Riesmeijer SA, Holt-Kedde IL, Werker PMN, Piersma B, Olinga P, Bank RA. Verteporfin ameliorates fibrotic aspects of Dupuytren's disease nodular fibroblasts irrespective the activation state of the cells. Sci Rep. 2022;12:13940. https://doi.org/10.1038/s41598-022-18116-9.
55. Kuhn MA, Wang X, Payne WG, Ko F, Robson MC. Tamoxifen decreases fibroblast function and downregulates TGF(beta2) in dupuytren's affected palmar fascia. J Surg Res. 2002;103:146–52. https://doi.org/10.1006/jsre.2001.6350.
56. Shih B, Bayat A. Scientific understanding and clinical management of Dupuytren disease. Nat Rev Rheumatol. 2010;6:715–26. https://doi.org/10.1038/nrrheum.2010.180.
57. Ulrich D, Hrynyschyn K, Pallua N. Matrix metalloproteinases and tissue inhibitors of metalloproteinases in sera and tissue of patients with Dupuytren's disease. Plast Reconstr Surg. 2003;112:1279–86. https://doi.org/10.1097/01.PRS.0000081462.40448.49.
58. Wilkinson JM, Davidson RK, Swingler TE, Jones ER, Corps AN, Johnston P, Riley GP, Chojnowski AJ, Clark IM. MMP-14 and MMP-2 are key metalloproteases in Dupuytren's disease fibroblast-mediated contraction. Biochim Biophys Acta. 2012;1822:897–905. https://doi.org/10.1016/j.bbadis.2012.02.001.
59. Layton T, Nanchahal J. Recent advances in the understanding of Dupuytren's disease. F1000Res. 2019;8:231. https://doi.org/10.12688/f1000research.17779.1.
60. Major M, Freund MK, Burch KS, Mancuso N, Ng M, Furniss D, Pasaniuc B, Ophoff RA. Integrative analysis of Dupuytren's disease identifies novel risk locus and reveals a shared genetic etiology with BMI. Genet Epidemiol. 2019;43:629–45. https://doi.org/10.1002/gepi.22209.
61. Majeed M, Wiberg A, Ng M, Holmes MV, Furniss D. The relationship between body mass index and the risk of development of Dupuytren's disease: a Mendelian randomization study. J Hand Surg Eur. 2021;46:406–10. https://doi.org/10.1177/1753193420958553.

62. Kim SK, Khan C, Ladd AL, Tashjian RZ. A shared genetic architecture between adhesive capsulitis and Dupuytren disease. J Shoulder Elb Surg. 2023;32:174–85. https://doi.org/10.1016/j.jse.2022.07.005.
63. Kuo RYL, Ng M, Prieto-Alhambra D, Furniss D. Dupuytren's disease predicts increased all-cause and cancer-specific mortality: analysis of a large cohort from the U.K. Clinical practice research Datalink. Plast Reconstr Surg. 2020;145:574e–82e. https://doi.org/10.1097/PRS.0000000000006551.
64. Bogdanov I, Rowland Payne C. Dupuytren contracture as a sign of systemic disease. Clin Dermatol. 2019;37:675–8. https://doi.org/10.1016/j.clindermatol.2019.07.027.
65. Ganesan S, Tantone RP, Komatsu DE, Hurst LC. The prevalence of Dupuytren's disease in patients with diabetes mellitus. Commun Med (Lond). 2023;3:96. https://doi.org/10.1038/s43856-023-00332-7.
66. Saini D, Kochar A, Poonia R. Clinical correlation of diabetic retinopathy with nephropathy and neuropathy. Indian J Ophthalmol. 2021;69:3364. https://doi.org/10.4103/ijo.IJO_1237_21.
67. Kovacs D, Demian L, Babeş A. Prevalence and risk of dupuytrèn disease in patients with diabetes versus non-diabetic patients. Rom J Diabetes Nutr Metab Dis. 2012;19:373–80. https://doi.org/10.2478/v10255-012-0043-z.
68. Abate M, Schiavone C, Salini V, Andia I. Occurrence of tendon pathologies in metabolic disorders. Rheumatology (Oxford). 2013;52:599–608. https://doi.org/10.1093/rheumatology/kes395.
69. Broekstra DC, Groen H, Molenkamp S, Werker PMN, van den Heuvel ER. A Systematic Review and Meta-Analysis on the Strength and Consistency of the Associations between Dupuytren Disease and Diabetes Mellitus, Liver Disease, and Epilepsy. Plast Reconstr Surg. 2018;141:367e–79e. https://doi.org/10.1097/PRS.0000000000004120.
70. Rydberg M, Zimmerman M, Löfgren JP, Gottsäter A, Nilsson PM, Melander O, Dahlin LB. Metabolic factors and the risk of Dupuytren's disease: data from 30,000 individuals followed for over 20 years. Sci Rep. 2021;11:14669. https://doi.org/10.1038/s41598-021-94025-7.
71. Takase F, Mifune Y, Inui A, Ueda Y, Kataoka T, Kokubu T, Kuroda R. Association of advanced glycation end products in Dupuytren disease. J Orthop Surg Res. 2018;13:143. https://doi.org/10.1186/s13018-018-0848-4.
72. Yuen A, Laschinger C, Talior I, Lee W, Chan M, Birek J, Young EWK, Sivagurunathan K, Won E, Simmons CA, McCulloch CA. Methylglyoxal-modified collagen promotes myofibroblast differentiation. Matrix Biol. 2010;29:537–48. https://doi.org/10.1016/j.matbio.2010.04.004.
73. Arafa M, Noble J, Royle SG, Trail IA, Allen J. Dupuytren's and Epilepsy Revisited. J Hand Surg. 1992;17:221–4. https://doi.org/10.1016/0266-7681(92)90095-J.
74. Skoog T. Dupuytren's contracture: pathogenesis and surgical treatment. Surg Clin North Am. 1967;47:433–44. https://doi.org/10.1016/s0039-6109(16)38187-7.
75. Critchley EM, Vakil SD, Hayward HW, Owen VM. Dupuytren's disease in epilepsy: result of prolonged administration of anticonvulsants. J Neurol Neurosurg Psychiatry. 1976;39:498–503. https://doi.org/10.1136/jnnp.39.5.498.
76. Tripoli M, Cordova A, Moschella F. Dupuytren's contracture as result of prolonged administration of phenobarbital. Eur Rev Med Pharmacol Sci. 2011;15:299–302.
77. Ling RS. The genetic factor in dupuytren's disease. J Bone Joint Surg Br. 1963;45:709–18.
78. James JIP. The relationship of Dupuytren's contracture and epilepsy. Hand. 1969;1:47–9. https://doi.org/10.1016/0072-968X(69)90040-0.
79. Murrell GAC. The role of the fibroblast in Dupuytren's contracture. Hand Clin. 1991;7:669–80. https://doi.org/10.1016/S0749-0712(21)00905-7.
80. Hindocha S, McGrouther DA, Bayat A. Epidemiological evaluation of Dupuytren's disease incidence and prevalence rates in relation to etiology. Hand. 2009;4:256–69. https://doi.org/10.1007/s11552-008-9160-9.
81. Wagner ER, Gottschalk MB, Karzon AL, Graf AR, O'Shaughnessy MA, Suh N. Dupuytren disease: surgical tips, optimizing outcomes, and cost considerations. Instr Course Lect. 2023;72:567–76.

82. Ng M, Lawson DJ, Winney B, Furniss D. Is Dupuytren's disease really a "disease of the Vikings"? J Hand Surg Eur. 2020;45:273–9. https://doi.org/10.1177/1753193419882851.
83. Saboeiro AP, Porkorny JJ, Shehadi SI, Virgo KS, Johnson FE. Racial distribution of Dupuytren's disease in department of veterans affairs patients. Plast Reconstr Surg. 2000;106:71–5.
84. Alser OH, Kuo RYL, Furniss D. nongenetic factors associated with Dupuytren's disease: a systematic review. Plast Reconstr Surg. 2020;146:799–807. https://doi.org/10.1097/PRS.0000000000007146.
85. Hindocha S. Risk factors, disease associations, and Dupuytren diathesis. Hand Clin. 2018;34:307–14. https://doi.org/10.1016/j.hcl.2018.03.002.
86. Mathieu S, Naughton G, Descatha A, Soubrier M, Dutheil F. Dupuytren's disease and exposure to vibration: systematic review and meta-analysis. Joint Bone Spine. 2020;87:203–7. https://doi.org/10.1016/j.jbspin.2020.02.001.
87. Al-Qattan MM. Factors in the pathogenesis of Dupuytren's contracture. J Hand Surg [Am]. 2006;31:1527–34.
88. Ke Q, Costa M. Hypoxia-inducible factor-1 (HIF-1). Mol Pharmacol. 2006;70:1469–80. https://doi.org/10.1124/mol.106.027029.
89. Holzer LA, Cör A, Pfandlsteiner G, Holzer G. Expression of VEGF, its receptors, and HIF-1α in Dupuytren's disease. Acta Orthop. 2013;84:420–5. https://doi.org/10.3109/17453674.2013.814011.
90. Türker T, Murphy E, Kaufman CL, Kutz JE, Meister EA, Hoying JB. Response of Dupuytren fibroblasts to different oxygen environments. J Hand Surg Am. 2013;38:2365–9. https://doi.org/10.1016/j.jhsa.2013.08.122.
91. Mayerl C, Del Frari B, Parson W, Boeck G, Piza-Katzer H, Wick G, Wolfram D. Characterisation of the inflammatory response in Dupuytren's disease. J Plast Surg Hand Surg. 2016;50:171–9. https://doi.org/10.3109/2000656X.2016.1140054.
92. McCarty S, Syed F, Bayat A. Role of the HLA system in the pathogenesis of Dupuytren's disease. Hand. 2010;5:241–50. https://doi.org/10.1007/s11552-009-9255-y.
93. Si Z, Wang X, Sun C, Kang Y, Xu J, Wang X, Hui Y. Adipose-derived stem cells: sources, potency, and implications for regenerative therapies. Biomed Pharmacother. 2019;114:108765. https://doi.org/10.1016/j.biopha.2019.108765.
94. Verhoekx JSN, Mudera V, Walbeehm ET, Hovius SER. Adipose-derived stem cells inhibit the contractile myofibroblast in Dupuytren's disease. Plast Reconstr Surg. 2013;132:1139–48. https://doi.org/10.1097/PRS.0b013e3182a3bf2b.
95. Ziegler ME, Staben A, Lem M, Pham J, Alaniz L, Halaseh FF, Obagi S, Leis A, Widgerow AD. Targeting myofibroblasts as a treatment modality for Dupuytren disease. J Hand Surg Am. 2023;48:914–22. https://doi.org/10.1016/j.jhsa.2023.06.007.

Chapter 3
Needle Aponeurotomy: Background and Technique

Yibo Li, Michael Lapner, and Armin Badre

3.1 History and Current Usage

Needle aponeurotomy, also known as percutaneous needle fasciotomy, uses a hypodermic needle to percutaneously release the cords causing Dupuytren's contracture. First described as a treatment for Dupuytren's disease by Sir Henry Cline [8], it was modified and popularized by French rheumatologists Lermusiaux and Debeyre in 1979 [25]. A French surgeon, Dr. Foucher, brought the technique to hand surgery in 2001 [16] and subsequently to the United States in 2003.

Notably, needle aponeurotomy has been found to be the most cost-effective treatment for Dupuytren's disease, both in the United States and Canadian healthcare systems [3, 23]. Despite the high recurrence rate after needle aponeurotomy [47], patients are satisfied and willing to undergo revision needle aponeurotomy for recurrence, which is equally safe to perform based on published literature [43, 44, 46].

3.2 Indications and Contraindications

Needle aponeurotomy is indicated in cooperative patients with a palpable cord causing contracture [13]. There are no universally accepted degrees of joint contractures meeting indications for treatment with needle aponeurotomy. While some authors advocate initiating treatment once an MCP joint contracture reaches over 30° or any degree of a PIP joint contracture has developed [11], others believe that any degree of symptomatic contracture can be an indication for needle aponeurotomy given its

Y. Li · M. Lapner · A. Badre (✉)
Western Hand & Upper Limb Facility, University of Alberta, Edmonton, AB, Canada
e-mail: badre@ualberta.ca

M. B. Gottschalk et al. (eds.), *Dupuytren's Disease*,
https://doi.org/10.1007/978-3-031-85873-4_3

low morbidity and risk profile [15, 35]. Generally, a shared decision-making model is employed as each patient has different thresholds of contracture tolerance. Given the minimally invasive nature and lower recurrence rate in older patients [43, 44], it is a safe option in the elderly who may have comorbidities placing them at higher risk from complications with a general anesthetic.

An absolute contraindication to needle aponeurotomy is no palpable cord [13]. Additionally, if a cord is not causing a contracture or the surgeon cannot tension the cord, then the patient is a poor candidate for the procedure. Relative contraindications include flap coverage or scarring over the planned surgical site, which increases the risk of neurovascular injury.

Rarely, a patient may present with severe flexor tendon bowstringing from prior injury or iatrogenesis which may mimic a cord. The surgeon should distinguish bowstringing from a cord by taking a careful history, examining the contracture (a flexor tendon glides under the fingers during finger range of motion while a cord does not), and/or using ultrasound.

Patients should be counseled preoperatively that PIP joint contracture is less amenable to correction with needle aponeurotomy due to capsular contracture, attenuation of the extensor tendon central slip, as well as abnormal thickened fascia along the lateral digital sheets, which may be difficult to access percutaneously [20, 22]. Furthermore, displacement of neurovascular bundles by spiral cords at this level increases the risk of neurovascular injury.

3.3 Training for Needle Aponeurotomy

The authors recommend that surgeons interested in performing needle aponeurotomy receive training by a hand surgeon familiar with the technique given the potential for neurovascular and flexor tendon injury, the high reliance on tactile feedback, and the steep learning curve. The authors recommend releasing easily palpable pretendinous cords, then progressing to more distal cords as comfort level increases when first implementing this technique.

3.4 Preoperative Planning

3.4.1 Anatomy

Pretendinous cords result in MCP joint contracture, central cords in PIP joint contracture, lateral cords in PIP or DIP joint contracture, natatory cords in webspace contracture, and spiral cords in PIP joint contracture [27]. The term “spiral cord” is a misnomer, as the cord itself becomes straight in Dupuytren’s disease and causes the digital neurovascular bundle to spiral and displace superficial and midline, creating a “spiral nerve” [39]. A detailed diagram of affected cords can be documented preoperatively (Fig. 3.1).

Dupuytren Evaluation: Office

Surname	Given Name
Date (dd/mm/yy) (/ /)	ID #

History

Age_______ Gender ☐M ☐F Writing Hand ☐R ☐L ☐B Dupuytren Hand ☐R ☐L ☐B

Age at diagnosis_______ Prior treatment ☐Y ☐N Age at first treatment_______

Treatment Details:

History of: Ledderhose ☐Y ☐N Frozen Shoulder ☐Y ☐N Peyronie ☐Y ☐N

Family history of Dupuytren or Ledderhose ☐Parents ☐Siblings ☐Other ☐None ☐Unknown

Family history details:

Other Relevant History:

Examination

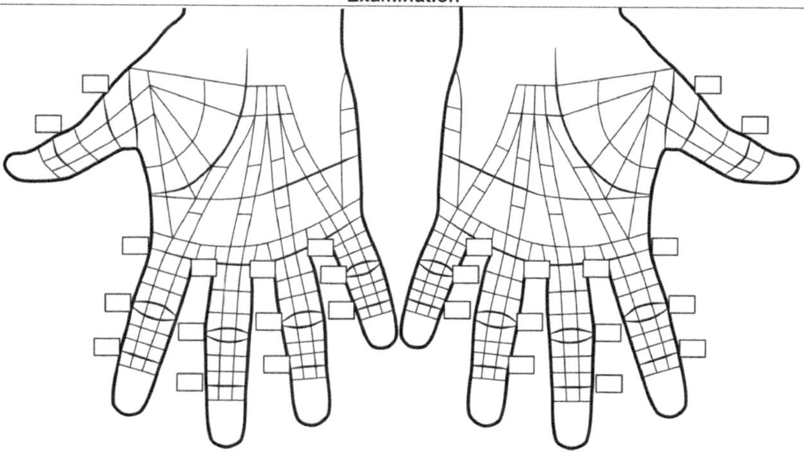

Mark the diagram using this legend:

☐ Extension Deficit ⁄⁄ Cord ※ Nodule ◇ Skin Involvement ⁝⁝ Skin Graft + Scar Ⓢ Doppler Spiral Bundle

	RIGHT	LEFT
Palmaris Longus	☐Present ☐Absent ☐Unknown	☐Present ☐Absent ☐Unknown
Doppler	☐No Exam ☐Normal ☐Inaudible ☐Spiral	☐No Exam ☐Normal ☐Inaudible ☐Spiral
Dorsal PIP Nodule	☐None ☐T ☐I ☐M ☐R ☐S	☐None ☐T ☐I ☐M ☐R ☐S
Additional Notes:		

Examiner:	Signature:

Fig. 3.1 Documentation form for preoperative examination of Dupuytren's contracture. (Reprinted with permission from the Dupuytren Research Group https://dupuytrens.org/wp-content/uploads/2023/06/2023-Dupuytren-Evaluation-Office-Version.pdf)

3.4.2 *Ultrasound Guidance*

Preoperative ultrasound mapping can be performed to identify the location of the arterial and neurologic supply to the palm and fingers, which can be marked with ink [37]. Ultrasound guidance is especially useful for spiral cords [13], given their tendency to displace the neurovascular bundles. While the use of ultrasound-guided needle aponeurotomy is safe with satisfactory results [30], no comparative studies exist to demonstrate the added value of ultrasound to routine needle aponeurotomy.

3.5 Technique

A video demonstration of the technique can be found at https://youtu.be/tscb5OPirwA.

3.5.1 *Setting and Equipment*

The procedure may be performed under wide-awake local anesthesia no tourniquet (WALANT) conditions in an office setting. The local anesthetic cocktail may include a combination of short- or long-acting local anesthetic, epinephrine, steroid, and sodium bicarbonate. The authors' preferred materials include towels, gauze, antiseptic preparation, and alcohol wipes; 1% lidocaine with epinephrine, sodium bicarbonate, and 40 mg of triamcinolone/methylprednisolone; a 30-gauge needle on a 5 mL syringe; an 18-gauge needle; and dressings (Fig. 3.2). Needle size varies among authors, with recommendations ranging from 25-gauge [10, 31, 35, 41, 43, 44], to 23-gauge [6] to 19-gauge [24] to 18-gauge [17]. The authors prefer an 18-gauge needle as its larger caliber makes it stiff enough to avoid bending throughout the procedure, it remains sharp, and it provides excellent tactile feedback.

3.5.2 *Preoperative Evaluation and Counseling*

Before starting the procedure, examine the affected digits visually to assess the degree of MCP, PIP, and DIP joint contracture. Palpate the cords to be treated and determine the planned portal sites. Portal sites should only be placed over palpable cords, not nodules (Fig. 3.3). Informed consent and allergies are reviewed. Counsel the patient that a skin tear may occur, often at the site of a needle aponeurotomy portal, and can be managed with local wound care and healing by secondary intention (see "Complications" section). The patient is warned that while the needle

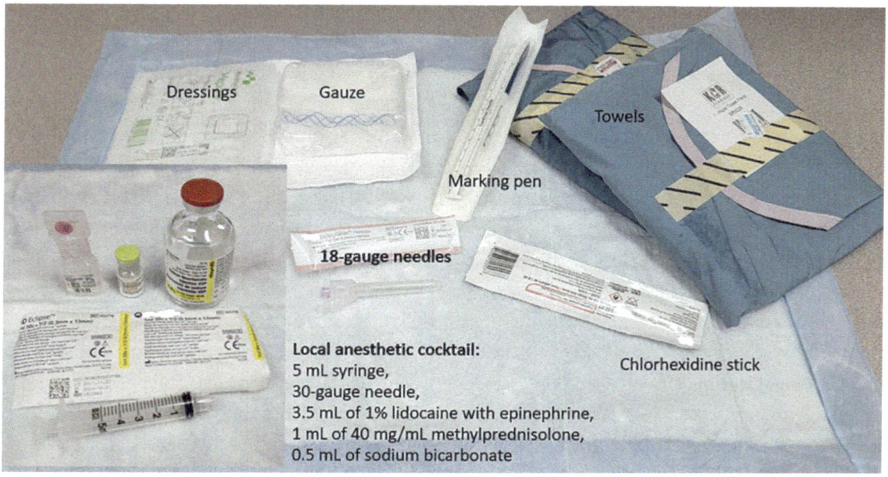

Fig. 3.2 Materials required for needle aponeurotomy

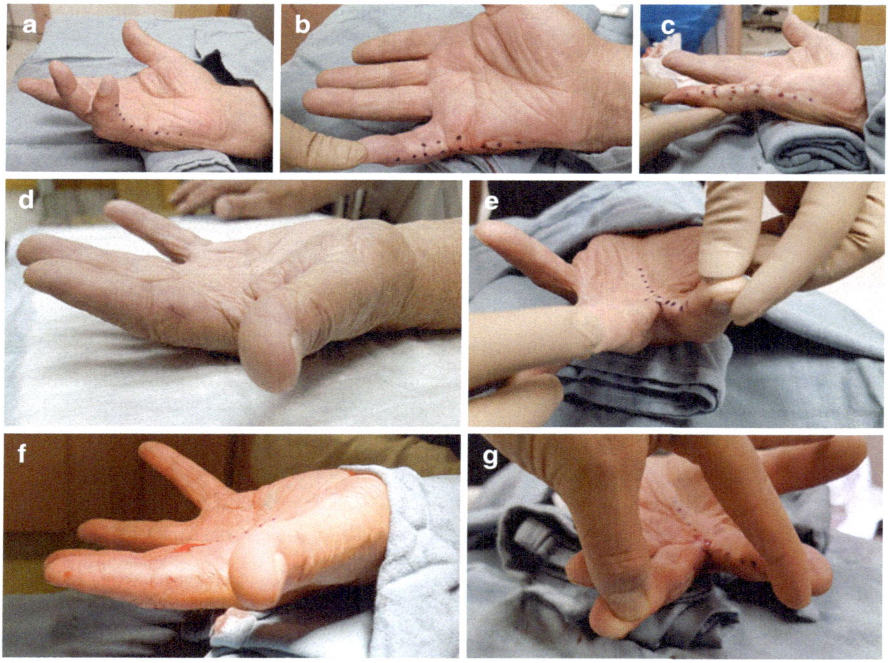

Fig. 3.3 (**a** and **b**) Planned portal sites along an abductor digiti minimi cord and a small finger lateral cord. Note the two side-by-side portals along the length of wide cords. (**c**) After needle aponeurotomy. (**d** and **e**) Planned portal sites along pretendinous and natatory cords of the same patient's contralateral hand. (**f** and **g**) After needle aponeurotomy

aponeurotomy portion of the procedure should not be painful, injection of local anesthetic and manipulation of the hand may be painful. The authors recommend avoiding digital blockade until later manipulation so that the patient can alert the surgeon when they experience paresthesias/severe pain, which indicate proximity of the needle to the digital nerves/flexor tendons. The cords are insensate, but the vital structures (including joint capsules, digital nerves, and flexor tendon sheaths) are sensate. Therefore, open communication with the patient throughout the procedure allows the surgeon to adjust needle positioning. The patient is also instructed to avoid sudden movements to reduce the risk of neurovascular and tendon injury.

Patients who require anticoagulation are instructed to continue their medication(s) preoperatively. Postoperatively, patients are told to hold pressure over the portal sites and to change dressings as needed should bleeding occur. To date, the authors have not encountered any significant bleeding issues with this technique. The addition of epinephrine to the local anesthetic cocktail can also aid in prevention of bleeding.

For patients with bilateral disease amenable to needle aponeurotomy, we generally recommend proceeding with treatment of the worse side first. If the patient requests both to be treated at the same time, we counsel the patient that they may have difficulties with self-care for the first few days after the procedure, and that we may discuss re-scheduling the second side if a skin tear occurs on the first.

3.5.3 Anesthesia

We encourage the use of multimodal analgesia and recommend that the patient take acetaminophen and ibuprofen 30 min prior to the procedure. Other techniques including topical anesthetics or holding an ice pack over the hand for 10 min beforehand can also be used.

The patient's hand is prepped and draped in the appropriate manner and anesthesia is administered intradermally into planned needle aponeurotomy portal sites. The authors use a 5 mL syringe with 3.5 mL of 1% lidocaine with epinephrine, 0.5 mL of sodium bicarbonate, and 1 mL of 40 mg/mL triamcinolone or methylprednisolone, then use a 30-gauge needle to inject aliquots of 0.1 to 0.2 mL of the mixture from proximal to distal along the cord to be treated. The local anesthetic may be injected along the planned portal sites all at once, or sequentially from proximal to distal. Additional local anesthetic may be used to supplement pain control throughout the procedure.

The patient's distal sensation is checked after infiltration of local anesthetic and throughout the procedure; if the finger becomes numb, the surgeon should proceed with caution and monitor the patient at follow-up for recovery, or abandon the procedure, particularly over higher risk areas such as a spiral cord, as the patient is no longer able to provide feedback regarding needle proximity to nerves.

3.5.4 *Patient Positioning*

The patient may be seated or lying supine with the affected hand on a hand table. A rolled-up towel is positioned underneath the hand to accentuate the cords by extension of the MCP and PIP joints. The surgeon should ensure adequate tension of the cord being treated using their non-dominant hand while handling the needle for aponeurotomy with their dominant hand, especially as the cord is sequentially released. However, the surgeon should note that when the pretendinous cord is progressively released and lengthened, the flexor tendons are at increased risk of injury as they bowstring superficially. To counteract this bowstringing, tension should be localized over the skin rather than applied to the entire finger, thereby keeping the flexor tendons relaxed. Additionally, the authors believe it is important to avoid inserting the needle deeper than the depth of its bevel to avoid lacerating the tendons, especially when new to the technique.

The flexor tendons will not bowstring to the same degree in the fingers due to the pulley system, and therefore passive extension of the finger while working on cords in the fingers is safe.

3.5.5 *Portal Placement*

Portals should generally be spaced 5–10 mm apart along the entire course of each cord to allow for adequate contracture correction. Sometimes, it is necessary to space portal sites more closely at 2–3 mm apart, such as when a cord is still palpable after release and the needle is too deep. Two side-by-side portals can be used for broad cords (Fig. 3.3). Placement of portals over flexion creases, at the base of the finger, or over an area of skin dimpling should be avoided, as skin tears are more likely to occur in these areas (Fig. 3.4). Also avoid placing a portal over an area of blanching, as this indicates tight skin rather than the presence of an underlying cord [13]. Once a cord is adequately released, the blanching will cross the previous area of cord contracture, indicating there is no more cord to release [13]. Furthermore, the presence of a spiral nerve can be predicted by a 2 cm soft, pulpy, compressible mass halfway between the distal palmar confluence and the proximal finger crease in the setting of PIP joint contracture [39]; these areas should also be avoided.

The authors recommend working from proximal to distal as it is easier to access the palm in cases of more severe contractures, though others describe beginning distal to allow the surgeon to move more proximal if the distal digital nerve accidentally becomes anesthetized [11, 14].

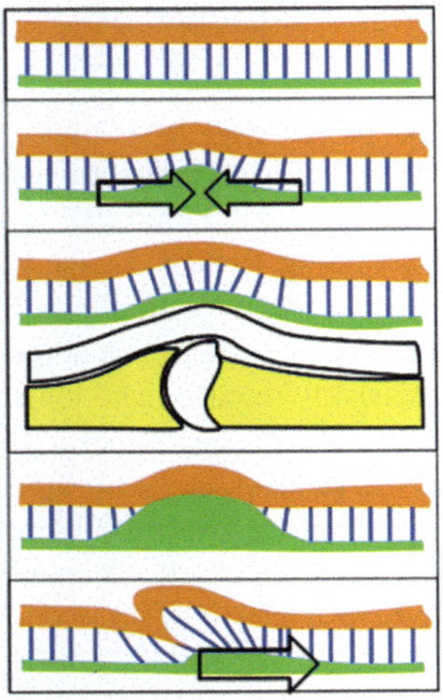

Fig. 3.4 Relevant anatomy to portal placement. (Reproduced with permission from [14], https://dupuytrens.org/DupPDFs/2010_Eaton.pdf)

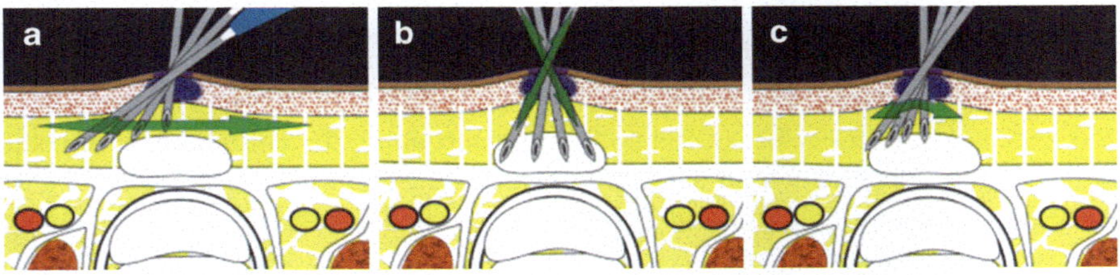

Fig. 3.5 (**a**) Clear: the bevel of the needle can be used to create a plane between the dermis and the cord. (**b**) Perforate: multiple shallow perforations can be performed through the same portal site while angling the needle in difference directions in a fan-shaped pattern. (**c**) Sweep: a sweeping, windshield wiper motion is used to divide cords during needle aponeurotomy. (Reproduced with permission from [12])

3.5.6 Needle Handling

The motion used to release each cord is a sweeping, windshield wiper motion (Figs. 3.5 and 3.6). It is important not to insert the needle too deeply within the cord, which would make it impossible to perform the sweeping motion. The needle should be inserted vertically to the surface of the cord, then swept radially and ulnarly over the cord. Prior to the sweeping motion, the bevel of the needle can be used to create a plane between the dermis and the cord (Fig. 3.5). When the cords are placed under sufficient tension by the surgeon's non-dominant hand extending the affected finger, a scraping sound followed by a sudden release of the contracture usually accompanies each release. A first superficial pass should be followed by cord palpation; if residual disease is palpable, then repeat the process through the same portal site more deeply.

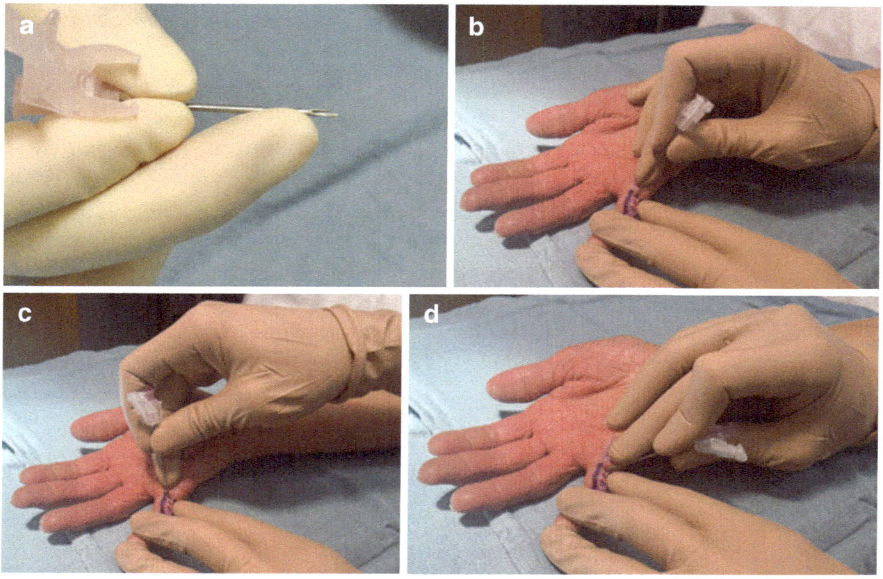

Fig. 3.6 How to hold the needle. (**a**) Notice the modified pencil grip, with the surgeon's long finger supporting the needle just proximal to the bevel. The surgeon's long finger is used as a brace against the patient's hand to avoid inserting the needle beyond the depth of its bevel. (**b**, **c**, and **d**) A windshield wiper motion is used to release the cord

To control needle insertion depth and thereby minimize risk of flexor tendon laceration, the authors recommend holding the needle like a pencil and using the surgeon's long finger as a brace against the patient's hand to prevent inserting the needle tip deeper than its bevel (Fig. 3.6). Moreover, multiple shallow perforations can be performed through the same portal site while angling the needle in different directions in a fan-shaped pattern to gain a better understanding of the depth and surface geometry of the cord (Fig. 3.5). This can be accomplished by first piercing the skin with a larger bore needle and then performing multiple passes through the cord with a smaller needle. Alternatively, other authors recommend attaching a syringe to the needle and using the syringe as a handle [36]. Regardless of the technique used, tactile feedback, both from the resistance of the cords on the needle tip and repeated palpation of remaining cords, is key to preventing injury to surrounding structures. The authors recommend releasing nearly the entire cord with needle aponeurotomy, then disrupting the remaining cord through manipulation. Another described technique to avoid flexor tendon injury involves inserting the needle and then asking the patient to flex and extend their PIP and DIP joints; motion of the needle indicates it is inserted into the flexor tendon [13].

The needle should be replaced once it no longer feels crisp when cutting, but rather feels rubbery when being inserted or withdrawn [13].

3.5.7 Special Cords

For abductor digiti minimi cords, care must be taken as the ulnar neurovascular bundle is in close proximity. Open communication with the patient, careful assessment of the cord, and judicious depth control of needle insertion are key. For natatory cords, the needle should be oriented perpendicular to the cord, which may be 90 degrees to the longitudinal axis of the finger (Fig. 3.7); massaging these cords may often help with release. Tensioning the natatory cords can be achieved by spreading the patient's affected fingers apart at the distal phalanges using the surgeon's index finger and thumb (Fig. 3.3g). For lateral and spiral cords leading to PIP joint contracture, the surgeon should use a narrower windshield wiper motion in order to stay on the cord and should closely communicate with the patient to avoid neurovascular injury.

3.5.8 Manipulation

Once the majority of a cord has been released with needle aponeurotomy, local anesthetic is injected as a digital block to facilitate manipulation; distal sensation is assessed beforehand as this injection usually results in whole fingertip numbness. The finger should be manipulated into extension to release the remainder of the cord. The surgeon's thumb can also be used to disrupt the cord by gently massaging

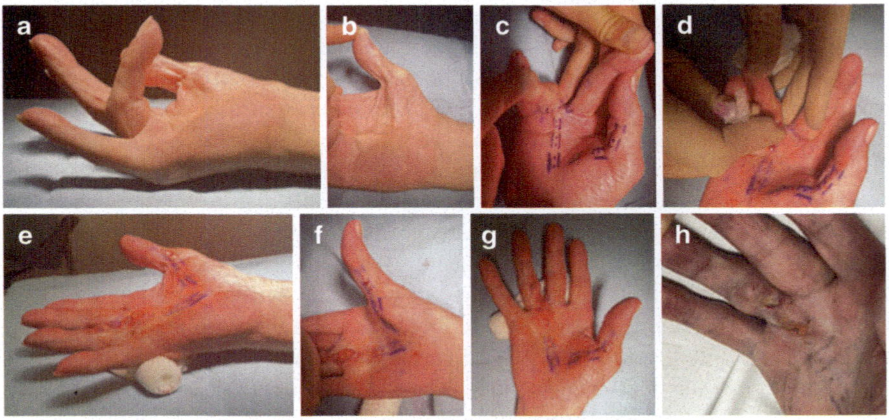

Fig. 3.7 (**a**, **b**, and **c**). Preoperative photos and planned portal sites demonstrating pretendinous and central cords to the ring finger leading to severe MCP and PIP joint contractures, thenar cord to the thumb leading to MCP joint contracture, and natatory cord in the third webspace leading to adduction contracture. (**d**) Needle aponeurotomy with the needle oriented longitudinally along the natatory cord, 90 degrees to the longitudinal axis of the finger. (**e**, **f**, and **g**) Postoperative photos showing correction of contractures and development of a skin tear. (**h**) Progressive healing of the skin tear at 2 weeks postoperatively

it in a longitudinal direction, especially for natatory and narrow lateral cords [35]. The patient is then asked to actively flex and extend their fingers to assess integrity of the flexor tendons.

If a skin tear occurs prior to manipulation, the authors recommend further releasing the cord at a different portal or performing subcision (see "Subcision" section) prior to manipulation to minimize the risk of propagating the tear. Further tips to minimize chances of a skin tear during manipulation include flexing the wrist to relax the flexor tendons; asking the patient to actively extend the finger at the same time; first extending the PIP joint with the MCP joint flexed and vice versa, then extending both joints together; and pulling on the skin distal to the portal in a proximal direction [14].

3.6 Postoperative Care

Bleeding should be controlled with direct pressure. Small adhesive dressings are applied over the portal sites; the dressing may be reinforced with a gauze wrap if there is persistent bleeding. Patients are instructed to extend their fingers actively and passively and to avoid strenuous activity for 1 week. At the conclusion of the case, it is helpful for the surgeon to instruct the patient on how to stretch and hold each digit that has been released into maximal extension. Specifically, the authors suggest the patient extend and hold each digit for 10–15 s with their contralateral hand, every 30–60 min during the day while awake. This becomes part of the patient's daily routine until follow-up to maintain the improvement obtained during the procedure.

Patients are seen at 10–14 days after the procedure to assess digital nerve function, maintenance of contracture correction, and wound healing. For patients without skin tears, follow-up is then as needed. Patients with skin tears are monitored until wounds are healed (Fig. 3.8).

We do not routinely splint the hand after needle aponeurotomy as it has not been shown to improve active range of motion of the MCP or PIP joints [42]. Further higher quality studies are required to corroborate this finding. We also do not routinely prescribe therapy after needle aponeurotomy.

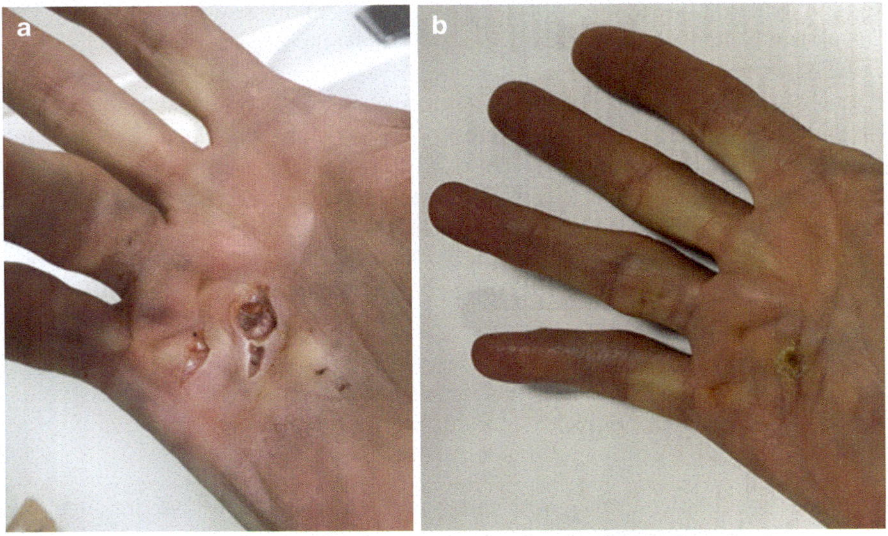

Fig. 3.8 Skin tear complicating needle aponeurotomy, immediately after needle aponeurotomy. Six weeks after the procedure, the patient's wounds healed uneventfully with dressing changes by secondary intention

3.7 Adjuncts

3.7.1 Steroid

Combining steroid injection with needle aponeurotomy has been shown to significantly reduce severity of total active extension deficit at mid-term follow-up and reduce likelihood of needing retreatment at 24 months [29]. Dosages of steroid injection vary in the literature as studies have combined different amounts of steroid in varying volumes of injection fluid. In a randomized controlled trial, McMillan et al. injected 8–48 mg of triamcinolone per digit immediately after needle aponeurotomy and at 6 weeks and 3 months after [28, 29]. Other authors report injecting steroid into the portal sites after release from preparations containing 5–6.7 mg/mL of triamcinolone [13, 15], or 10–13.3 mg/mL of methylprednisolone prior to aponeurotomy [35, 41]. Our injection fluid contains 8 mg/mL of triamcinolone or methylprednisolone which is injected into planned portal sites before needle aponeurotomy to minimize spillage of steroid from widened post-release portal sites.

3.7.2 Percutaneous Aponeurotomy and Lipofilling (PALF)

First introduced in 2011 and updated in 2015 [18, 19], PALF involves making dozens of shallow punctures with a 19-gauge needle along the entire length of the palpable cord, followed by injection of 10 mL of gravity-sedimented lipoaspirate through 2–3 needle entry sites in the palm and digit [19]. The liposuction donor area is typically the abdomen [19]. In theory, the adipose-derived-stem cells in the lipoaspirate inhibit contractile myofibroblast proliferation [45]; furthermore, fat grafting is thought to restore the subdermal fat deficiency and atrophy associated with Dupuytren's disease [19]. Patients are splinted for up to 1 week postoperatively [19]. Although randomized controlled trial data has shown that PALF resulted in significantly shorter rehabilitation time with similar operative contracture correction compared to limited fasciectomy [21], five-year recurrence rate is significantly higher [38]. Furthermore, there are no trials directly comparing needle aponeurotomy to PALF. The benefit of lipofilling is therefore unclear and is not routinely performed by the authors.

3.7.3 *Subcision*

Originally described by Adams [2], subcision involves the use of a needle to release vertical fibers connecting the cords to the skin, thereby mobilizing any tethered skin (pitting) or creases [34]. This technique has been described for the treatment of any depressed cutaneous scars or wrinkles [34]. When performing subcision, the needle should be as parallel to the skin as possible to avoid damage to critical structures [9], and the bevel should be facing superficially [34]. Similar to needle aponeurotomy, the needle should be swept side-to-side to release pitting. Subcision can also be used to release the attachments of the Cleland and Grayson ligaments at the lateral PIP joint [9].

3.8 Complications

Skin tears are the most common complication after needle aponeurotomy, and have been reported in 3.4–68% of cases [1, 17, 33, 35, 36]. Patients with more severe preoperative contracture are warned of a higher risk of skin tear; these usually occur over portal sites, creases, and areas of skin dimpling. Although they can appear severe, sometimes with exposed tendon and neurovascular structures, skin tears heal well by secondary intention and require no intervention other than local wound care (Fig. 3.8).

Although often cited as a potential complication, flexor tendon injury is rare, with most series reporting no ruptures [16, 33, 35]. Patients are instructed to make a fist at the end of the procedure to verify the integrity of the tendon. If a laceration occurs, the tendon can be immediately repaired under wide-awake, local anesthesia, no tourniquet (WALANT) technique.

Digital nerve injury occurs in 0.1% of cases [35]. If identified during the procedure, a digital nerve repair may be performed concurrently under local anesthesia. However, if the digital nerves are inadvertently anesthetized during the procedure and identification of the nerve injury is delayed until the first postoperative follow-up visit, repair within 14 days is also associated with excellent outcomes [26]. More commonly, a neuropraxia can occur which resolves by 3 months [1, 35, 36].

Digital artery injury with needle aponeurotomy is extremely rare [7]. The finger may however appear ischemic due to injection of local anesthetic and/or from vasospasm [7]. The patient is instructed to observe the finger over the following hours and to return to clinic if the appearance does not resolve spontaneously. Persistent ischemia is treated with phentolamine injection [32].

Infection occurs in up to 0.7% of cases [4, 17] and can be treated with oral antibiotics if superficial and irrigation and debridement if deep.

3.9 Recurrence

Recurrent disease should be expected after needle aponeurotomy, with a rate of 50–85% reported at 5 years [5, 43, 44]. Well-developed recurrent cords are most amenable to revision needle aponeurotomy, whereas recurrent contracture from diffuse scarring and fibrosis without a clear cord often require open procedures [22]. Revision needle aponeurotomy is safe and effective and can be performed recurrently, resulting in similar rates of contracture correction up to the fourth recurrence [43, 44, 46].

References

1. Abe Y, Tokunaga S. Clinical results of percutaneous needle fasciotomy for Dupuytren's disease in Japanese patients. Plast Reconstr Surg Glob Open. 2015;3(5):e384. https://doi.org/10.1097/GOX.0000000000000338.
2. Adams W. Observations on contraction of the fingers (Dupuytren's contraction) and its successful treatment by subcutaneous divisions of the palmar fascia, and immediate extension, vol. 1. London: Churchill; 1879. p. 928.
3. Baltzer H, Binhammer PA. Cost-effectiveness in the management of Dupuytren's contracture: a Canadian cost-utility analysis of current and future management strategies. Bone Joint J. 2013;95-B(8):1094–100. https://doi.org/10.1302/0301-620X.95B8.31822.
4. Beaudreuil J, Lellouche H, Orcel P, Bardin T. Needle Aponeurotomy in Dupuytren's disease. Joint Bone Spine. 2012;79(1):13–6. https://doi.org/10.1016/j.jbspin.2011.03.003.
5. Chen N, Srinivasan R, Shauver M, Chung K. A systematic review of outcomes of fasciotomy, aponeurotomy, and collagenase treatments for Dupuytren's contracture. Hand. 2011;5(3):250–5.
6. Cheng HS, Hung LK, Tse WL, Ho PC. Needle aponeurotomy for Dupuytren's contracture. J Orthop Surg (Hong Kong). 2008;16(1):88–90. https://doi.org/10.1177/230949900801600120.
7. Cheung K, Walley KC, Rozental TD. Management of complications of Dupuytren contracture. Hand Clin. 2015;31(2):345–54. https://doi.org/10.1016/j.hcl.2015.01.005.
8. Cline H. Notes on pathology. London: St Thomas Hospital Medical School Library; 1777.
9. Denkler KA, Vaughn CJ, Dolan EL, Hansen SL. Evidence-based medicine: options for Dupuytren's contracture: incise, excise, and dissolve. Plast Reconstr Surg. 2017;139(1):240e–55. https://doi.org/10.1097/PRS.0000000000002857.

10. Denkler KA, Park KM, Alser O. Treatment options for Dupuytren's disease: tips and tricks. Plast Reconstr Surg Glob Open. 2022;10(1):e4046. https://doi.org/10.1097/PRS.0000000000009641.
11. Diaz R, Curtin C. Needle aponeurotomy for the treatment of Dupuytren's disease. Hand Clin. 2014;30(1):33–8. https://doi.org/10.1016/j.hcl.2013.09.005.
12. Eaton C. Evidence-based medicine: Dupuytren contracture. Plast Reconstr Surg. 2014;133(5):1241–51. https://doi.org/10.1097/PRS.0000000000000089.
13. Eaton C. Percutaneous fasciotomy for Dupuytren's contracture. J Hand Surg Am. 2011;36(5):910–5. https://doi.org/10.1016/j.jhsa.2011.02.016.
14. Eaton C. Needle aponeurotomy: terminology and methodology; 2010. https://dupuytrens.org/DupPDFs/2010_Eaton.pdf
15. Elzinga KE, Morhart MJ. Needle aponeurotomy for Dupuytren disease. Hand Clin. 2018;34(3):331–44. https://doi.org/10.1016/j.hcl.2018.03.003.
16. Foucher G, Medina J, Malizos K. Percutaneous needle fasciotomy in Dupuytren disease. Tech Hand Up Extrem Surg. 2001;5(3):161–4. https://doi.org/10.1097/00130911-200109000-00007.
17. Herrera FA, Mitchell S, Elzik M, Roostaeian J, Benhaim P. Modified percutaneous needle aponeurotomy for the treatment of Dupuytren's contracture: early results and complications. Hand. 2015;10(3):433–7. https://doi.org/10.1007/s11552-015-9740-4.
18. Hovius SER, Kan HJ, Smit X, Selles RW, Cardoso E, Khouri RK. Extensive percutaneous aponeurotomy and lipografting: a new treatment for Dupuytren disease. Plast Reconstr Surg. 2011;128(1):221–8. https://doi.org/10.1097/PRS.0b013e31821741ba.
19. Hovius SER, Kan HJ, Verhoekx JSN, Khouri RK. Percutaneous aponeurotomy and lipofilling (PALF). Clin Plast Surg. 2015;42(3):375–81. https://doi.org/10.1016/j.cps.2015.03.006.
20. Hovius SER, Zhou C. Advances in minimally invasive treatment of Dupuytren disease. Hand Clin. 2018;34(3):417–26. https://doi.org/10.1016/j.hcl.2018.03.010.
21. Kan HJ, Selles RW, Van Nieuwenhoven CA, Zhou C, Khouri RK, Hovius SER. Percutaneous Aponeurotomy and Lipofilling (PALF) versus limited Fsciectomy in patients with primary Dupuytren's contracture: a prospective, randomized, controlled trial. Plast Reconstr Surg. 2016;137(6):1800–12. https://doi.org/10.1097/PRS.0000000000002224.
22. Kaplan FTD, Crosby NE. Treatment of recurrent Dupuytren disease. Hand Clin. 2018;34(3):403–15. https://doi.org/10.1016/j.hcl.2018.03.009.
23. Leafblad ND, Wagner E, Wanderman NR, Anderson GR, Visscher SL, Kremers HM, Larson DR, Rizzo M. Outcomes and direct costs of needle aponeurotomy, collagenase injection, and Fasciectomy in the treatment of Dupuytren contracture. J Hand Surg Am. 2019;44(11):919–27. https://doi.org/10.1016/j.jhsa.2019.07.017.
24. Lee MVK, Hunter-Smith D. Needle fasciotomy for Dupuytren's disease: an Australian perspective. ANZ J Surg. 2009;79(11):776–8. https://doi.org/10.1111/j.1445-2197.2009.05101.x.
25. Lermusiaux JL, Debeyre N. L'actualité Rhumatologique 1979 Présentée Aux Praticien. Paris: Expansion Scientifique Francaise; 1980.
26. MacKay BJ, Cox CT, Valerio IL, Greenberg JA, Buncke GM, Evans PJ, Mercer DM, McKee DM, Ducic I. Evidence-based approach to timing of nerve surgery: a review. Ann Plast Surg. 2021;87(3):e1–21. https://doi.org/10.1097/SAP.0000000000002767.
27. McFarlane RM. Patterns of the diseased fascia in the fingers in Dupuytren's contracture. Plast Reconstr Surg. 1974;54(1):31–44.
28. McMillan C, Binhammer P. Steroid injection and needle aponeurotomy for Dupuytren contracture: a randomized, controlled study. J Hand Surg Am. 2012;37(7):1307–12. https://doi.org/10.1016/j.jhsa.2012.04.026.
29. McMillan C, Binhammer P. Steroid injection and needle aponeurotomy for Dupuytren disease: long-term follow-up of a randomized controlled trial. J Hand Surg Am. 2014;39(10):1942–7. https://doi.org/10.1016/j.jhsa.2014.07.018.
30. Molenkamp S, Van Straalen RJM, Werker PMN, Broekstra DC. Imaging for Dupuytren disease: a systematic review of the literature. BMC Musculoskelet Disord. 2019;20(1):224. https://doi.org/10.1186/s12891-019-2606-0.

31. Morhart M. Pearls and pitfalls of needle aponeurotomy in Dupuytren's disease. Plast Reconstr Surg. 2015;135(3):817–25. https://doi.org/10.1097/PRS.0000000000000961.
32. Nodwell T. How long does it take phentolamine to reverse adrenaline-induced vasoconstriction in the finger and hand? A prospective, randomized, blinded study: the Dalhousie project experimental phase. Can J Plast Surg. 2003;11(4)
33. Nydick JA, Olliff BW, Garcia MJ, Hess AV, Stone JD. A comparison of percutaneous needle fasciotomy and collagenase injection for Dupuytren disease. J Hand Surg Am. 2013;38(12):2377–80. https://doi.org/10.1016/j.jhsa.2013.08.096.
34. Orentreich DS, Orentreich N. Subcutaneous incisionless (Subcision) surgery for the correction of depressed scars and wrinkles. Dermatologic Surg. 1995;21:543–9.
35. Pess GM. Tips and pearls for PNF and collagenase: a ten-year personal experience. In: Dupuytren disease and related diseases: the cutting edge. Switzerland: Springer; 2017. p. 161–70.
36. Rijssen AL, et al. A comparison of the direct outcomes of percutaneous needle fasciotomy and limited fasciectomy for Dupuytren's disease: a 6-week follow-up study. J Hand Surg Am. 2006;31(5):498.
37. Sakellariou VI, Brault J, Rizzo M. Ultrasound-assisted percutaneous needle fasciotomy for Dupuytren's contracture. Edited by Steven F. Harwin Orthop. 2015;38(5):299–303. https://doi.org/10.3928/01477447-20150504-03.
38. Selles RW, Zhou C, Kan HJ, Wouters RM, Van Nieuwenhoven CA, Hovius SER. Percutaneous aponeurotomy and lipofilling versus limited fasciectomy for Dupuytren's contracture: 5-year results from a randomized clinical trial. Plast Reconstr Surg. 2018;142(6):1523–31. https://doi.org/10.1097/PRS.0000000000004982.
39. Short WH, Kirk Watson H. Prediction of the spiral nerve in Dupuytren's contracture. J Hand Surg Am. 1982;7(1):84–6. https://doi.org/10.1016/S0363-5023(82)80020-8.
40. Soreide E, Murad MH, Denbeigh JM, Lewallen EA, Dudakovic A, Nordsletten L, van Wijnen AJ, Kakar S. Treatment of Dupuytren's contracture. Bone Joint J. 2018;100(9):1138.
41. Strömberg J. Percutaneous needle fasciotomy for Dupuytren contracture. JBJS Essent Surg Tech. 2019;9(1):e6. https://doi.org/10.2106/JBJS.ST.18.00047.
42. Tam L. Needle aponeurotomy for Dupuytren contracture: effectiveness of postoperative night extension splinting. Plast Surg. 2016;24(1):23.
43. Rijssen V, Annet L, Ter Linden H, Werker PMN. Five-year results of a randomized clinical trial on treatment in Dupuytren's disease: percutaneous needle fasciotomy versus limited fasciectomy. Plast Reconstr Surg. 2012a;129(2):469–77. https://doi.org/10.1097/PRS.0b013e31823aea95.
44. Rijssen V, Annet L, Werker PMN. Percutaneous needle fasciotomy for recurrent Dupuytren disease. J Hand Surg Am. 2012b;37(9):1820–3. https://doi.org/10.1016/j.jhsa.2012.05.022.
45. Verhoekx JSN, Mudera V, Walbeehm ET, Hovius SER. Adipose-derived stem cells inhibit the contractile myofibroblast in Dupuytren's disease. Plast Reconstr Surg. 2013;132(5):1139–48. https://doi.org/10.1097/PRS.0b013e3182a3bf2b.
46. Vlot MA, Werker PMN. Effectiveness of percutaneous needle fasciotomy for second or higher recurrence in Dupuytren contracture. In: Dupuytren disease and related diseases: the cutting edge. Switzerland: Springer; 2017. p. 179–84.
47. Werker PMN, Pess GM, Van Rijssen AL, Denkler K. Correction of contracture and recurrence rates of Dupuytren contracture following invasive treatment: the importance of clear definitions. J Hand Surg Am. 2012;37(10):2095–2105.e7. https://doi.org/10.1016/j.jhsa.2012.06.032.

Chapter 4
Needle Aponeurotomy: Evidence-Based Outcomes

Kitty Y. Wu

4.1 Introduction

Percutaneous fasciotomy for the management of Dupuytren's contracture was first described by Sir Astley Paston Cooper in 1822 [1]. Cooper used a long thin bisotry blade to percutaneously transect the thickened palmar fascia to correct flexion deformities [1]. This was later refined in 1797 by French rheumatologists Lermusiaux and Debeyre who used a needle, instead, to perform the fasciotomy [2, 3]. However, it would be more than 20 years later that percutaneous needle aponeurotomy (NA) would be introduced in North America by Dr. Charles Eaton at the 2003 annual American Society for Surgery of the Hand meeting. Since then, there has been a resurgence in the use of NA. This technique offers a minimally invasive, office-based procedure that can be performed under local anesthesia (Fig. 4.1a–d). Many patients are able to obtain almost complete correction of their flexion contractures (Fig. 4.1e, f) with limited downtime. This chapter provides an evidence-based review of the efficacy, recurrence rate, complications, cost-effectiveness, and patient-reported outcomes of needle aponeurotomy for the treatment of Dupuytren's disease (Table 4.1).

K. Y. Wu (✉)
Plastic and Hand Surgeon, Mayo Clinic, Rochester, MN, USA
e-mail: wu.kitty@mayo.edu

M. B. Gottschalk et al. (eds.), *Dupuytren's Disease*,
https://doi.org/10.1007/978-3-031-85873-4_4

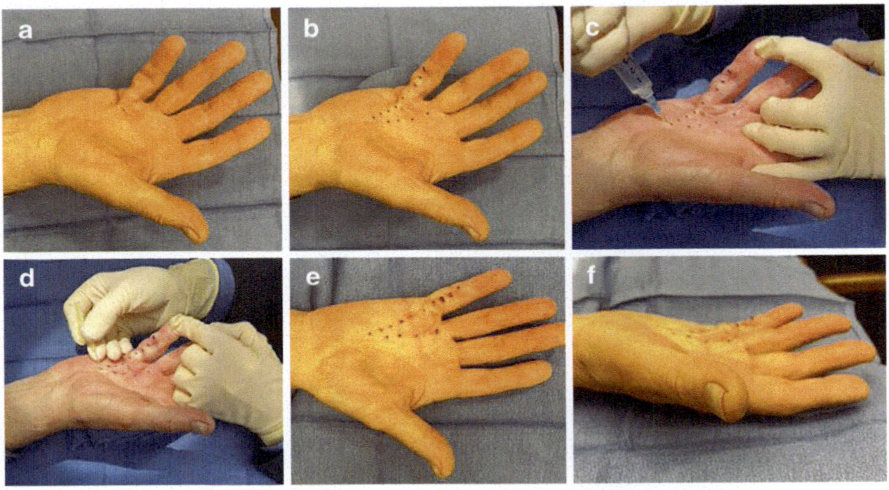

Fig. 4.1 Needle aponeurotomy for primary Dupuytren's contracture. A 75-year-old male presented with primary Dupuytren's disease of his right small finger, resulting in 80° MCPJ and 25° PIPJ contractures (**a**). Needle aponeurotomy was performed as an office-based procedure under local anesthesia (**b**, **c**). Aponeurotomy was performed at 1 cm intervals using a 19 gauge needle in the palm and 22 gauge needle in the finger (**d**). Immediate results following the procedure demonstrate full extension at the PIPJ and within 5° of full extension at the MCPJ (**e**, **f**). (Case courtesy of Marco Rizzo)

Table 4.1 Outcomes of needle aponeurotomy

Article	Number of digits	Mean baseline contracture (°)		Immediate following NA (°)		Final follow-up (°)		Recurrence rate (%)		Mean follow-up
		MCP	PIP	MCP	PIP	MCP	PIP	MCP	PIP	
Van Rijssen et al. [6]	88	44	34	17[a]	24[a]	9	21			6 weeks
Pess et al. [7]	1013	35	50	1	6	11	35	20	65	3 years
Van Rijssen et al. [5]	93	43	35					84.9		5 years
Herrera et al. [20]	525	30	33	< 1	2	24	19			4.5 months
Stromberg et al. [10]	71	46	7	−4[a]		0		1.4		1 years
Zhou et al. [23]	78	38	19			10	18	24		12 weeks
Leafblad et al. [21]	367	34.1	31.5					24 (2 year); 61 (5 year)		5 years
Zachrisson et al. [11]	58	45	48	10	26	0	30	29.3		6.5 years
Denkler et al. [14]	204	70	75			10	45			22.3 months
Abe et al. [22]	48	38	43			13	9.4–26	29		3 years
NA with adjuncitive procedures										
Selles et al. [32] (lipofilling)	31	21	39			24	47	21 (1 year); 74 (5 year)		5 years
McMillan et al. [27] (steroid injection)	44	101 TPED				34 TPED				4.4 years
NA for recurrent contractures										
Van Rijssen et al. [16]	40	50 TPED				13 TPED		50		4.4 years

[a]1-week post procedure; *TPED* total passive extension deficit

4.2 Expected Outcomes

Clinical success in the management of Dupuytren's disease is most often defined as achieving within 5° of full extension in the affected digit [4–6]. In one of the largest patient cohorts, Pess et al. reviewed over 1000 digits treated with NA. These patients had mean baseline MCPJ and PIPJ contractures of 35° and 50°, respectively. Immediately following NA, 99% of MCPJ contractures and 89% PIPJ contractures were corrected to within 5° of full extension [7]. At three-year follow-up, this correction was maintained in 72% of MCPJ, but only 31% of PIPJ. Numerous studies demonstrate that the results for the correction of MCPJ flexion contractures are superior to the PIPJ for all treatment strategies, including NA [4, 5, 7–9]. With finger flexion, the collateral ligaments of the MCPJ are lengthened, while they are shortened for the PIPJ and DIPJ. With prolonged flexed posturing of the affected digit, the collateral ligaments contract and fasciotomy alone may not fully correct the deformity.

Van Rijssen et al. examined the early results of patients at 1 and 6 weeks after NA and demonstrated the ongoing improvement of MCPJ, but not PIPJ, contractures [4]. In this review of 166 digits, the mean reduction of MCPJ total passive extension deficit (TPED) at 1 week was 67%, which increased to 75% at 6 weeks. For the PIPJ, however, the TPED at 1 week was 34% at 1 week and 33% at 6 weeks [4]. A different study found that these immediate results can be maintained in the long term. A Swedish study of 71 patients showed that 90% of patients had reduction of MCPJ contractures (to less than 5°) at 1 week following treatment, and this was maintained at 1 year after injection [10].

Longer term follow-up of van Rijssen et al.'s initial study showed that the correction of flexion contractures was maintained in 55% of MCPJ and only 26% of PIPJ at 5 years [5]. When stratified by age, patients over the age of 55 had greater success in maintaining their result and a lower rate of recurrence. Older patients may have less aggressive disease with a slower rate of progression, while younger patients presenting for treatment may have faster progressing disease and Dupuytren's diasthesis. A smaller cohort study of NA in 58 digits with 6.5-year follow-up showed that the mean TPED of 52° at baseline was reduced to 20° post-procedure. At the final follow-up, the TPED at 23° [11] demonstrates that, in some patients, these results can be stable in the long term.

Beaudreuil et al. examined the results of patients receiving multi-needle aponeurotomy (MNA), where four or more treatments were administered at a single visit, targeted either at multiple digits or multiple locations on a single digit [12]. The immediate outcomes in 37 patients and 99 digits showed almost complete correction (mean 2.6° extension lag) at the MCPJ. Outcomes were worse at the PIPJ, with a mean post-procedure extension lag of 22.7° [12]. At 6 months, there was slight increase in the flexion deformity at both joints (9.5° at MCPJ, and 28.4% at the PIPJ); however, 95% of patients reported satisfaction with their outcomes [12].

4.2.1 Severe Contractures

From van Rijssen et al's 2006 study, patients with higher grades of flexion contracture, based on the Tubiana grade (Table 4.2) [13], had worse results following NA [4]. Patients with Tubiana Grade 1 or II disease (less than 90° flexion contractures)

Table 4.2 Tubiana grade

Grade	Total passive extension deficit
I	0° to 45°
II	45° to 90°
III	90° to 135°
IV	≥ 135°

had a 67–71% reduction of TPED; whereas Grade III or IV patients (greater than 90° flexion contractures) had a 46–47% reduction of TPED. Denkler and Park reported their outcomes of 165 patients, including 204 digits, with severe Dupuytren's disease. This was defined as patients with greater than 135° of total combined passive extension loss of the MCPJ, PIPJ, and DIPJ [14]. NA was still effective in this group with 74% improvement in MCPJ contractures (70° TPED pre-procedure to 10° post-procedure) and 32% improvement in PIPJ contractures (75° TPED pre-procedure to 45° post-procedure). While this still marks a significant improvement, these results are worse compared to patients in other studies with less severe disease [5–7].

4.2.2 *Recurrent Disease*

Needle aponeurotomy can also be an effective treatment option for patients with recurrent disease (Fig. 4.2). In a systematic review of treatment modalities for recurrent Dupuytren's contracture, including 12 studies and 224 affected digits, 56.6% of patients were treated with fasciectomy [15]. However, the second most common treatment modality, in 21.9% of patients, was NA [15]. In a study of 30 patients with recurrent disease treated with NA, there was a 93% reduction of TPED at the MCPJ and 57% reduction at the PIPJ [16]. At a mean of 4.4 years follow-up, 50% of patients remained free of secondary recurrence, defined as an increase of more than 30° of flexion contracture compared to their previous baseline. The other 50% of patients reported recurrence at a mean of 1.4 years after treatment, and all were managed without complication by limited fasciectomy. In a follow-up study, the results of NA for third, fourth, and fifth time recurrences were reported in 16 digits. Patients undergoing third or fourth NA treatments had a 73% and 63% reduction in TPED. By the fifth treatment with NA, there was a sharp decline to only a 27% reduction of TPED [17]. NA can be considered in patients presenting with recurrent disease; however, the efficacy sharply declines beyond four repeated treatments.

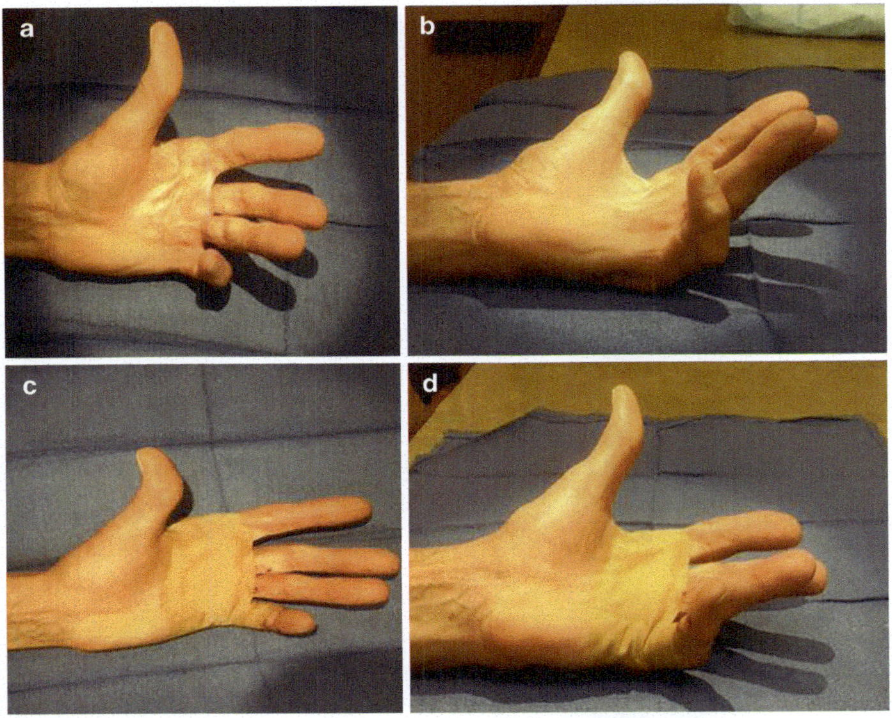

Fig. 4.2 Needle aponeurotomy for recurrent Dupuytren's contracture. A 72-year-old male patient presented with Dupuytren's contractures in his left ring and small fingers (**a**, **b**). He underwent prior limited fasciectomy 2 years ago and reports achieving full extension in both digits. He now presents with recurrent disease and 50° MCPJ and 57° PIPJ contractures in the small finger. Needle aponeurotomy was performed under local anesthesia in an office-based setting at 1 cm intervals along the palpable cords. Immediate results following the procedure (**c**, **d**) show mild correction of the MCPJ and PIPJ contractures. (Case courtesy of Marco Rizzo)

4.3 Recurrence Rates

The direct comparison of recurrence rates between studies is difficult owing to the varying definitions of recurrence in the literature. In a systematic review of 218 English studies on the management of Dupuytren's disease, there were 21 different definitions of recurrence [18]. Furthermore, in the majority of these studies, recurrence was defined qualitatively. Using each individual study's definition of recurrence, the overall reported recurrence rate for NA was 33–100% [18]. Commonly used quantitative definitions of recurrence include a passive extension deficit of greater than 30° [6] or a return of more than 20° of contracture in previously successfully treated joints [19].

Dupuytren's disease is not curable, and with enough time, patients will invariably have natural continued progression or "return" of disease, regardless of the treatment option. Therefore, the timing of follow-up assessments will also influence the reported recurrence rates. A large series of 525 digits treated with NA reported a recurrence rate of 12% at a mean of 4-month follow-up [20]. As expected, with increasing time from procedure, the reported recurrence rates similarly increased. A systematic review performed in 2011 reported a recurrence rate of 50–58% for NA at a mean follow-up time of 3–5 years [8]. In a recent randomized control trial of 93 patients with 5-year follow-up, the recurrence rate was 84.9% at 5 years [5]. Recurrence also occurred earlier in the NA group, reported as early as 6 months post-treatment compared to 2 years in patients who underwent open fasciectomy [5]. A different study reported that the reintervention rate for NA was 24% at 2 years and 61% at 5 years [21]. There is also a higher reported rate of recurrence for the PIPJ compared to the MCPJ. Abe et al 's study showed that, at 3-year follow-up of a group of 34 patients, there was a 29% recurrence rate for the MCPJ and 60% for the PIPJ [22]. Greater severity of PIPJ contractures was found to be predictive of need for earlier re-intervention [21]. These recurrence rates are similar or slightly higher compared to collagenase injections; however, significantly higher compared to open limited fasciectomy techniques [4, 15, 21, 23–26].

4.4 Adjunctive Techniques

In addition to needle fasciotomy, adjuncts such as the addition of steroid medication and autologous fat grafting have been proposed to help improve outcomes. In one randomized control trial, patients either underwent NA alone or NA with steroid injection. Patients received 8–48 mg of triamcinolone per digit, based on severity, administered at the time of NA and at 6 weeks and 3 months post-procedure. At 6 months, the triamcinolone group had greater correction of their flexion deformity (13% residual active extension deficit compared to 36% in the NA-only group) [27]. In a follow-up study, the added benefit of the triamcinolone injection was maintained up to 24 months; however, after 2 years, there was no difference in mean total active extension deficit between the two groups [27].

The addition of autologous fat grafting with NA has been proposed to improve both the aesthetic appearance of the hand and as a potential method of reducing contracture recurrence. There is growing literature to support the regenerative and anti-fibrotic effects of adipose-derived stem cells, especially in the post-radiation setting [28, 29]. Hovius et al. reported on 50 patients where 10 mL of autologous fat was injected subcutaneously after NA was performed. 95% of patients were very satisfied with the results, subjectively reporting a more supple appearance of the hand. In this group, there was a mean decrease in TPED of 37° to −5° for MCP contractures and of 61° to 27° in PIPJ contractures; however, there was no comparative group of patients with NA alone [30]. A 2015 prospective randomized study comparing percutaneous aponeurotomy and lipofilling (PALF) to limited fasciectomy demonstrated a similar degree of contracture correction and no difference in recurrence at 1 year [31]. While neither of these studies directly compared PALF to

NA alone, the typical results of NA underperform limited open fasciectomy and therefore the equivalent results of PALF with fasciectomy are encouraging. These results, however, were not maintained in the long term. At 5 5-year follow-up of this same cohort, there was a 74% recurrence rate in the PALF group compared to 39% in limited fasiectomy [32]. Furthermore, PALF is performed under regional or general anesthesia, whereas NA alone can be an office-based procedure requiring only local anesthesia. Future randomized, comparative, long-term studies between NA and PALF are required to determine if the added benefits of autologous fat grafting outweigh the costs, time, and risks of anesthesia.

4.4.1 Complication Rates

The overall complication rates following NA are significantly lower compared to both collagenase injections and open fasciectomy [33]. Major complications following needle aponeurotomy, such as acute or delayed flexor tendon rupture, digital nerve injury or transection, digital vascular compromise, flexor tenosynovitis, or complex regional pain syndrome (CRPS), are rare. In a Danish National Patient Registry study of 2257 patients with 3331 treated digits and 7.2-year median follow-up, the cumulative complication rate was 1.7% [34]. In terms of major complications, there were four patients (0.02%) with acute flexor tendon ruptures, and one patient (0.04%) with nerve transection, but no reported cases of CRPS. Another large Canadian series of 2000 digits treated with NA similarly showed a low overall complication rate with 5% incidence of skin tears, 2–5% risk of transient neuropraxia, 0.1% rate of acute flexor tendon rupture, and no permanent neurovascular injuries [33]. In this series, the reported incidence of temporary neurapraxia or transient paresthesias is between 1.2% and 5% [7, 33] and often resolves without any required intervention by 2–3 weeks post-procedure. The risk of complete nerve transection was lower and was reported between 0.04% and 2% [22, 34]. Risks of major infections requiring operative incision and debridement are also exceedingly rare, with only two cases of flexor tenosynovitis following NA reported in the literature [20].

The most common minor complications following NA are skin tears resulting from passive manipulation of the flexed digit, reported in 3.4–68% of cases [7, 20, 33]. The vast majority of these cases can be managed conservatively with dressings and wound care and skin grafting is rarely indicated or required. The most common areas of skin tears were at the base of the MCPJ and in places where the underlying cord is adherent to the skin. In these cases, needle subcision can be performed prior to releasing the cord. Performing multiple needle fasciotomies along the same cord prior to manipulation can also aid in decreasing the incidence of skin tears.

Complication rates are slightly higher in patients with severe Dupuytren's disease, defined as greater than 135° TPED [14]. In a series of 165 patients with severe disease, there was one patient who required amputation after skin graft loss and resulting osteomyelitis. Two patients experienced transient neurapraxia and one had partial digital nerve injury. The incidence of skin tears was 4%; however, most patients required skin grafting. This indicates that the size of skin tears is likely greater than in patients with less severe disease, where skin tears are most frequently managed conservatively. While patients with severe contractures can still be effectively treated with NA, this study indicates a slightly higher risk of major complications requiring operative intervention.

The use of ultrasound guidance with NA has been proposed as a method of visualizing the critical neurovascular structures in the digit to avoid injury. A study of US-guided NA in 70 digits reported a 6% rate of skin tears and minor hematomas, but no case of nerve, tendon, or vascular injury [35]. Another study using modified high-frequency ultrasound guidance for NA in 42 patients demonstrated good results with no reported flexor tendon ruptures or neurovascular injuries [36].

4.5 Cost-Effectiveness

NA has been shown in numerous studies to be cost-effective compared to open fasciectomy from both the societal and patient perspective. Based on cost-effective analysis using a traditional willingness-to-pay threshold of $50,000 per quality-adjusted life year (QALY), the cost of NA, per QALY, was 8.5 times less when compared to open partial fasciectomy [37]. A similar Canadian study also identified NA as the most cost-effective strategy from a societal perspective for the treatment of patients with primary and recurrent Dupuytren's contracture in a single digit [38]. From a patient perspective, another study compared direct costs (surgical, anesthesia, and facility fees) in 48 patients undergoing either open fasciectomy or NA in the United States. The mean patient cost of open fasciectomy was $11,240 (range $4061 to $20,915) compared to $4657 ($3910 to $6514) for NA. In another study from the United States, the estimated immediate direct costs of NA was $624 per digit and the cumulative cost was $1540 per digit at 5 years [21]. France, Maravic and Beaudreuil reported that replacing open fasciectomy with NA for patients with single-digit disease would reduce treatment costs by 90% and overall healthcare costs by 56–59% [39]. While the exact cost of NA differs around the world, it still remains the most cost-effective strategy for the treatment of Dupuytren's disease.

4.6 Patient Satisfaction

There are high rates of patient-reported satisfaction following needle aponeurotomy. In a Dutch study by Zhou et al, patients who underwent NA had higher reported satisfaction, improved activities of daily living, and better overall hand function compared to patients with limited fasciectomy [23]. In van Rijssen's 2012 study with 5-year follow-up, patients with NA were less satisfied than those with limited fasciectomy, and this was strongly negatively influenced by recurrent disease. However, 26 of 45 patients with recurrent disease still chose to undergo NA a second time, despite being offered other treatment options [5].

Kan et al explored patient preferences for the management of DD comparing NA, PALF, collagenase injections, and limited fasciectomy [40]. A total of 506 patients were surveyed in a discrete choice experiment where they had to repeatedly make choices between two treatment options, with adjusted hypothetical complication rates, recurrence rates, recovery times, and residual extension deficits. Overall, recurrence rate, residual extension deficit, and complication rate were the most important considerations for patients when deciding. Furthermore, patients indicated they would be willing to accept an 11% increased recurrence rate if they could receive NA instead of undergoing limited open fasciectomy.

In another mixed methods study of 30 participants, who have received treatment of Dupuytren's contracture, there was a high rate of satisfaction among all patients, regardless of treatment choice [41]. Patients who had prior limited fasciectomies were willing to undergo a more invasive procedure and extensive recovery time as a means for a longer-term solution. Comparatively, patients who underwent NA perceived these treatments as safer, more convenient, and allowing for more rapid return to work. This study emphasizes that, with a full discussion of the benefits and trade-offs of each procedure, high patient satisfaction can be achieved regardless of treatment choice.

4.7 Conclusions

Needle aponeurotomy offers a safe, minimally invasive, and effective treatment option for the management of primary and recurrent Dupuytren's contracture. Despite a higher rate of recurrence when compared to open fasciectomy, NA provides effective immediate and long-term correction of MCPJ and PIPJ contractures, even in patients with severe and recurrent disease. With high rates of patient satisfaction, needle aponeurotomy should be discussed and considered as a potential treatment option for patients with both primary and recurrent Dupuytren's contractures.

References

1. Hutchison RL, Rayan GM. Astley Cooper: his life and surgical contributions. J Hand Surg Am. 2011;36(2):316–20.
2. Lermusiaux JL, Debeyre N. Le traitement medical de la maladie de Dupuytren. In: de Seze S, Ryckewaert A, Kahn MF, Guerin CI, editors. L'actualite rhumatologique. Expansion Scientifique Franchaise; 1980. p. 338–843.
3. Badois FJ, Lermusiaux JL, Masse C, Kuntz D. Non-surgical treatment of Dupuytren disease using needle fasciotomy. Rev Rhum Ed Fr. 1993;60(11):808–13.

4. van Rijssen AL, Gerbrandy FSJ, Ter Linden H, Klip H, Werker PMN. A comparison of the direct outcomes of percutaneous needle fasciotomy and limited fasciectomy for Dupuytren's disease: a 6-week follow-up study. J Hand Surg Am. 2006;31(5):717–25.
5. van Rijssen AL, Ter Linden H, Werker PMN. Five-year results of a randomized clinical trial on treatment in Dupuytren's disease: percutaneous needle fasciotomy versus limited fasciectomy. Plast Reconstr Surg. 2012;129(2):469–77.
6. van Rijssen AL, Werker PMN. Percutaneous needle fasciotomy in dupuytren's disease. J Hand Surg Br. 2006;31(5):498–501.
7. Pess GM, Pess RM, Pess RA. Results of needle aponeurotomy for Dupuytren contracture in over 1,000 fingers. J Hand Surg Am. 2012;37(4):651–6.
8. Chen NC, Srinivasan RC, Shauver MJ, Chung KC. A systematic review of outcomes of fasciotomy, aponeurotomy, and collagenase treatments for Dupuytren's contracture. Hand. 2011;6(3):250–5.
9. Beaudreuil J, Lellouche H, Orcel P, Bardin T. Need for a standard procedure for needle aponeurotomy, consensus definition of recurrence, and functional assessment in dupuytren disease. Plast Reconstr Surg. 2012;130(1):200e–1e.
10. Stromberg J, Ibsen-Sorensen A, Friden J. Comparison of treatment outcome after collagenase and needle fasciotomy for Dupuytren contracture: a randomized, single-blinded, clinical trial with a 1-year follow-up. J Hand Surg Am. 2016;41(9):873–80.
11. Zachrisson A, Sorensen AI, Stromberg J. Needle fasciotomy for Dupuytren's contracture- a prospective cohort study of 58 fingers with a median follow-up of 6.5 years. J Plast Surg Hand Surg. 2020;54(2):89–93.
12. Beaudreuil J, Lermusiaux JL, Teyssedou JP, et al. Multi-needle aponeurotomy for advanced Dupuytren's disease: preliminary results of safety and efficacy (MNA 1 study). Joint Bone Spine. 2011;78(6):625–8.
13. Tubiana R. Surgical management. In: Tubiana R, editor. The hand. WB Saunders Company; 1999. p. 480.
14. Denkler KA, Park KM. Needle Aponeurotomy for stage IV Dupuytren contracture: a wide-awake first step approach in 204 consecutive rays. Plast Reconstr Surg. 2022;150(5):1033e–6e.
15. Wong CR, Huynh MNQ, Fageeh R, McRae MC. Outcomes of management of recurrent Dupuytren contracture: a systematic review and meta-analysis. Hand. 2022;17(6):1104–13.
16. van Rijssen AL, Werker PMN. Percutaneous needle fasciotomy for recurrent Dupuytren disease. J Hand Surg Am. 2012;37(9):1820–3.
17. Vlot MA, Werker PMN. Effectiveness of percutaneous fasciotomy for second or higher recurrence in Dupuytren's contracture. In: Werker PMN, Dias J, Eaton C, Reichert B, Wach W, editors. Dupuytren disease and related diseases: the cutting edge. Berlin: Springer; 2017. p. 179–84.
18. Werker PM, Pess GM, van Rijssen AL, et al. Correction of contracture and recurrence rates of Dupuytren contracture following invasive treatment: the importance of clear definitions. J Hand Surg Am. 2012;37(10):2095–105.
19. Badalamente MA, Hurst LC. Efficacy and safety of injectable mixed collagenase subtypes in the treatment of Dupuytren's contracture. J Hand Surg Am. 2007;32(6):767–74.
20. Herrera FA, Mitchell S, Elzik M, et al. Modified percutaneous needle aponeurotomy for the treatment of dupuytren's contracture: early results and complications. Hand. 2015;10(3):433–7.
21. Leafblad ND, Wagner E, Wanderman NR, et al. Outcomes and direct costs of needle aponeurotomy, collagenase injection, and fasciectomy in the treatment of Dupuytren contracture. J Hand Surg Am. 2019;44(11):919–27.
22. Abe Y. Comparison of treatment outcomes after collagenase injection and percutaneous needle fasciotomy for Dupuytren's contracture: objective and subjective comparisons with a 3-year follow-up. Plast Reconstr Surg. 2020;145(6):1464–74.
23. Zhou C, Selles RW, Slijper HP, et al. Comparative effectiveness of percutaneous needle aponeurotomy and limited fasciectomy for Dupuytren's contracture: a multicenter observational study. Plast Reconstr Surg. 2016;138(4):837–46.

24. Zhang D, Earp BE, Blazar P. Collagenase treatment versus needle fasciotomy for single-digit Dupuytren contractures: a meta-analysis of randomized controlled trials. J Hand Surg Am. 2023;48:1200.
25. Soreide E, Murad MH, Denbeigh JM, et al. Treatment of Dupuytren's contracture: a systematic review. Bone Joint J. 2018;100-B(9):1138–45.
26. Peimer CA, Blazar P, Coleman S, et al. Dupuytren contracture recurrence following treatment with collagenase clostridium histolyticum (CORDLESS [collagenase option for reduction of Dupuytren long-term evaluation of safety study]): 5-year data. J Hand Surg Am. 2015;40(8):1597–605.
27. McMillan C, Binhammer P. Steroid injection and needle aponeurotomy for Dupuytren disease: long-term follow-up of a randomized controlled trial. J Hand Surg Am. 2014;39(10):1942–7.
28. Truong JL, Liu M, Tolg C, et al. Creating a favorable microenvironment for fat grafting in a novel model of radiation-induced mammary fat pad fibrosis. Plast Reconstr Surg. 2020;145(1):116–26.
29. Borrelli MR, Diaz Deleon NM, Adem S, et al. Fat grafting rescues radiation-induced joint contracture. Stem Cells. 2020;38(3):382–9.
30. Hovius SER, Kan HJ, Smit X, et al. Extensive percutaneous aponeurotomy and lipografting: a new treatment for Dupuytren disease. Plast Reconstr Surg. 2011;128(1):221–8.
31. Hovius SE, Kan HJ, Verhoekx JS, et al. Percutaneous aponeurotomy and lipofilling (PALF): a regenerative approach to Dupuytren contracture. Clin Plast Surg. 2015;42(3):375–81. ix
32. Selles RW, Zhou C, Kan HJ, et al. Percutaneous aponeurotomy and Lipofilling versus limited fasciectomy for Dupuytren's contracture: 5-year results from a randomized clinical trial. Plast Reconstr Surg. 2018;142(6):1523–31.
33. Elzinga KE, Morhart MJ. Needle aponeurotomy for Dupuytren disease. Hand Clin. 2018;34(3):331–44.
34. Therkelsen LH, Skov ST, Laursen M, et al. Percutaneous needle fasciotomy in Dupuytren contracture: a register-based, observational cohort study on complications in 3,331 treated fingers in 2,257 patients. Acta Orthop. 2020;91(3):326–30.
35. Villanueva M, Iborra A, Fahandezh-Saddi H, et al. Ultrasound-guided aponeurotomy and interphalangeal joint capsular release for treatment of Dupuytren's disease. J Hand Surg Eur. 2022;47(7):742–9.
36. Mi S, Zhang X, Han M, et al. Modified dynamic high-frequency ultrasound-guided needle aponeurotomy for Dupuytren's contracture. Hand Surg Rehabil. 2021;40(5):637–42.
37. Chen NC, Shauver MJ, Chung KC. Cost-effectiveness of open partial fasciectomy, needle aponeurotomy, and collagenase injection for Dupuytren contracture. J Hand Surg Am. 2011;36(11):1826–34.
38. Baltzer H, Binhammer PA. Cost-effectiveness in the management of Dupuytren's contracture. A Canadian cost-utility analysis of current and future management strategies. Bone Joint J. 2013;95-B(8):1094–100.
39. Maravic M, Beaudreuil J. Impact on costs of switching one-ray aponeurectomy to percutaneous needle aponeurotomy in Dupuytren's disease: a model analysis. Joint Bone Spine. 2015;82(4):264–6.
40. Kan HJ, de Bekker-Grob EW, van Marion ES, et al. Patients' preferences for treatment for Dupuytren's disease: a discrete choice experiment. Plast Reconstr Surg. 2016;137(1):165–73.
41. Kane RL, Wood SM, Cichocki MN, et al. Evaluating shared decision-making in treatment selection for Dupuytren contracture: a mixed methods approach. Plast Reconstr Surg. 2023;151(2):255e–66e.

Chapter 5
Collagenase Injections: Background and Technique

Brianne J. Sullivan, Paul Marji, and Harvey Chim

5.1 Background

5.1.1 Introduction

Dupuytren's disease (DD) is a fibroproliferative disorder that affects the palmar aponeurosis and causes flexure contractures of the digits. The small and ring fingers are most frequently involved. Treatment is typically advised with flexion contracture of at least 30 degrees at the metacarpophalangeal (MCP) or proximal interphalangeal (PIP) joints [1]. Yet, the optimal time of intervention is debated, with some authors focusing more on the associated disability than the degree of flexion [5]. Surgical excision of the diseased tissue has been the gold standard treatment [2]. However, surgery can be costly and disease can recur. Surgery for DD has higher scar burden and potential for wound breakdown and infection and carries a risk for neurovascular injury. Thus, nonsurgical options have been explored that can be implemented in an office-based setting, decrease morbidity, decrease cost and recovery time, but still improve function and quality of life [3]. Collagenase Clostridium histolyticum (CCH) injections have become a popular nonsurgical treatment option that have shown excellent outcomes in properly selected patients [4].

B. J. Sullivan (✉) · P. Marji · H. Chim
Division of Plastic and Reconstructive Surgery, Louisiana State University Health Sciences Center, New Orleans, LA, USA

M. B. Gottschalk et al. (eds.), *Dupuytren's Disease*,
https://doi.org/10.1007/978-3-031-85873-4_5

5.1.2 Pharmacology

Seven collagenases have been isolated from the bacteria C. histolyticum. They are all zinc-dependent matrix metalloproteinases and hydrolyze collagen molecules via specific binding domains, allowing cleavage of the protein into short segments. They can be divided into two classes, I and II, which are categorized by their genetics and where they act on the collagen molecule. The breakdown of the molecule is a product of the two classes acting at multiple sites along the peptide chain. These collagenases remain active over a wide pH range, have a high degree of substrate specificity, lack autodigestion, lyophilize safely, and reconstitute providing easy storage and good stability. CCHs require Ca^{2+} ions to be active and need to be diluted in a buffer solution containing Ca^{2+} ions prior to use. CCHs are manufactured through bacterial fermentation, and even though the different collagenases can be separated chromatographically, the ratio and activity of class I and class II is challenging to control with this method and therefore can produce CCHs with varied biologic effects [3].

5.1.3 History

CCH is the first non-surgical, pharmacologic treatment available for Dupuytren's disease [6]. CCH functions by targeting collagen-based Dupuytren's disease cords while sparing the healthy surrounding tissue. The pathophysiology of DD is complicated, multifactorial, and not fully understood. At its foundation, there is excessive fibroblast proliferation, myofibroblast production, and collagen deposition that creates distinctive cords and nodules. Normal palmar fascia is mainly composed of type I collagen, while in DD there is an abundance of type III collagen. Collagen composes nearly 30% of all the proteins found in the human body. Collagen is an insoluble matrix protein consisting of three helical wound polypeptides and its triple helical nature makes it difficult to degrade [3].

Clostridium histolyticum is a clostridia species that was first discovered in the late nineteenth century. Its effect on collagen was not uncovered until the 1920s. In 1931 and 1932 it was reported that the anaerobe could digest small pieces of Achilles tendon [7]. A new isolated enzyme from C. histolyticum responsible for destroying the collagen framework was coined collagenase shortly after. In the 1960s and 1970s the use of "enzymatic fasciotomy" was employed during open surgery as well as via an injection using trypsin, hyaluronidase, and lidocaine [8]. In the early 1980s, a study was published examining the effect of CCH on human Peyronie disease tissue using rats to elucidate the dose necessary for collagenolysis. A subsequent rat study extrapolated cytotoxic doses in humans. Lethal doses were found to be hundreds of times higher than the doses required for collagenolysis at a local injection level [3].

In 1996, an in vitro study was performed looking at the effect of CCH on the tensile strength of DD cords, which demonstrated that a 300-unit dose of collagenase was able to achieve cord rupture [9]. In 2000, a phase II study investigated in-vivo efficacy and safety of CCH injections with 32 patients. Using the in vitro research as a guide, 300 U was initially injected into the cord, but this did not result in cord rupture, and the dose was incrementally increased until eventually 10,000 U of CCH was used successfully, with cord rupture achieved on passive digital extension the following day. Each patient showed correction of MCP and PIP contractures to 0–15 degrees in all but two patients, with no one sustaining any major adverse events. Minor adverse events included local irritation at injection site, tenderness, edema, small hematoma, and upper arm lymphadenopathy. This study also evaluated the immunogenic effects of CCH injections by following serum immunoglobulin E (Ig) assays. The participant's IgE titers did increase, but this was not found to have any clinical impact, and titers decreased with time from injection [10].

The same group of authors organized another Phase II, dual-phased, randomized, placebo-controlled, double-blinded trial in 2002 that compared the effect of a placebo, 5000 U, and 10,000 U CHC injection in patients with DD and MCP or PIP joint contractures [11, 12]. They established the optimal injection dose to be 10,000 U showing statistically significant outcomes in the degree of contracture compared to placebo and the lower dose. The secondary endpoint sought to elucidate changes in strength and range of motion with no significant loss seen in either group. Yet again, adverse events were minor with 3 patients experiencing skin tears from the rapid stretch with the extension maneuver. This study also evaluated CCH pharmacokinetics by checking serum and urine levels of collagenase up to 24 h after injection, which showed no collagenase in the serum and up to 28% of the dose collected from the urine, with no evidence of renal damage. The substudy additionally demonstrated that lidocaine injection prior to the extension maneuver did not negatively impact efficacy of the CHC injection [11].

Over the course of a decade, a handful of other studies evaluated CCH for DD, Peyronie disease, and hypertrophic scars [13, 14]. Badalamente and Hurst continued their research publishing a Phase III randomized, placebo-controlled, double-blinded trial in 2007 [4]. This study used 10,000 U of an original subtype of a CCH preparation on a total of 55 Dupuytren's contracture patients with similar outcomes for the primary endpoint of less than 5 degrees of contracture within 30 days of injection. Ninety-one percent of the contracted joints in the intervention group obtained clinical success compared to 0% in the placebo group. As before, no serious adverse events were seen and a two-year follow-up showed 5 joint recurrences—one MCPJ and four PIP joints.

Hurst et al. proceeded to publish the first level 1 evidence evaluating CCH injections for DD. The randomized control trial with 512 joints highlighted a clear benefit of a novel CCH preparation, called Xiaflex® (Auxilium Pharmaceuticals Inc., Malvern, PA), over placebo for flexion contractures secondary to DD (2009).

5.1.4 *Xiaflex®*

An original CCH designed specifically for medical applications with reproducible and consistent quantities of collagenase class ratios is marketed as Xiaflex® [3]. Xiaflex® was studied in vitro on PD and DD cords by Del Carlo [15]. This research showed enzymes were active within 4 h and had near complete breakdown of collagen by 12 h, without harming any noncollagenous tissue, regardless of the dose.

According to FDA.gov, Xiaflex was approved by the Federal Drug Administration (FDA) in 2010 for the treatment of adult patients with Dupuytren's contracture with a palpable cord at a dose of 0.58 mg/injection and 0.9 mg/vial [16]. The approved frequency of use is up to 3 injections per cord at 4-week intervals.

FDA approval of Xiaflex® was primarily based on two randomized, double-blind, placebo-controlled studies, CORD I and CORD II. There was a total of 374 people enrolled with metacarpophalangeal (MCP) contractures of 20–100 degrees and proximal interphalangeal (PIP) joint contractures of 20–80 degrees, with the primary endpoint looking for reduction in contracture to 5 degrees or less within 30 days of the treatment.

The Collagenase Option for the Reduction of Dupuytren's (CORD) I, the larger of the two trials, was funded by Auxilium Pharmaceuticals and had a sample size of 308 patients at 16 centers across the United States with 64% in the CHC group achieving the primary endpoint, compared to 6.8% in the placebo group [2].

The CORD II trial was based out of Australia and was also a double-blind, randomized, placebo-controlled study with 66 patients. They had the same primary endpoint with 44.4% success for the CHC injection and 4.8% with the placebo [17].

For the CORD studies, the patients were healthy and at least 18 years old. Patients who used anticoagulants within the past 7 days and who had MCP contracture over 100 degrees or PIP over 80 degrees were excluded. There was no recurrence at 90 days. Contracture less than 50 degrees portends a 90% chance of reducing contracture to under 5 degrees. Adverse events were reported by 96% of the collagenase cohort but events were mostly mild to moderate and resolved in 10 days without intervention. The most common complaints were swelling, bruising, itching, and pain in the injected hand. Three patients developed a treatment-related major adverse event, one case of complex regional pain syndrome and two tendon ruptures. Two of the ruptures were in cords associated with the PIP joint of the small finger (fda.gov). In line with surgical studies, Xiaflex® had greater success with MCP joint contracture than the PIP joint. Hand or orthopedic surgeons primarily administered the injections. At an average of 7 months, 4–11% of subjects noted recurrence. All subjects developed antibodies to collagenase, though none developed anaphylaxis [2].

5.1.5 *Current Trends*

Collagenase injections have now been a part of the accepted treatment plan for Dupuytren's disease for over a decade in the United States. During the first 3 years after FDA approval there were 26 tendon ruptures out of over 49,000 injections

(0.05%). Given the clinical scenario and frequency was similar to the initial clinical trials no safety-related changes were made to the product guidelines [6]. Nonetheless, 75% of the tendon ruptures occurred in the small finger and thus experts advocate to stay more proximal, not cross the finger crease, and to remain more superficial in the cord (va.gov) [12]. Xiaflex® was initially approved for a single injection of 0.58 mg every 4 weeks, for a total of three doses. Subsequently, two injections of 0.58 mg into multiple cords was shown to be safe [18]. The finger manipulation maneuver remains most commonly performed the day after the injection, but the MULTICORD study demonstrated that waiting 48 or 72 hours had a similar safety and efficiency profile and a trend toward less skin tears [6].

Five-year follow-up data after CCH injection showed a recurrent joint contracture of 47%, 39% at the MCP, and 66% at the PIP joints, with contracture defined as 20 degrees or more [19]. This is on par with the expected recurrence after open fasciotomy, which is roughly 30–50% [20]. Studies have shown collagenase injections are cost-effective, with the total treatment for a single patient being lower than an open fasciectomy if the patient requires one or two injections [21] [22]. Satisfaction rates are high, but these scores decrease as recurrence increases [23]. Sixty-seven percent of one cohort that underwent collagenase injection at least 5 years ago endorsed they would undergo treatment again, and another study of 213 patients 73% were satisfied or very satisfied after 3 years [24].

Authors have published on alternative techniques for Xiaflex® injection, primarily using a higher dose [25, 26] but most publications and practitioners follow the manufacturer's guidelines.

5.2 Technique

As per the manufacturer's guideline, Xiaflex® lyophilized powder must be reconstituted using the provided diluent prior to use, as it contains necessary calcium for enzyme activity. Before reconstitution, the drug needs to be removed from refrigeration and thawed at room temperature for 15–60 min. Each palpable Dupuytren's cord with a contracture in a metacarpophalangeal (MCP) joint or proximal interphalangeal (PIP) joint receives 0.58 mg of Xiaflex®. Up to two cords on the same hand can be treated per visit, using separate vials and syringes for each reconstitution and injection site [27].

Reconstitution involves a 1.0 mL syringe with 0.01 mL gradations and a 27-gauge ½ inch needle. The diluent should be slowly injected down the vial's side and gently swirled. The solution should be clear. If it is not clear it should not be injected. Local anesthetic before injection is discouraged, as it may interfere with proper placement of the Xiaflex® medication [27].

Greater amounts of diluent are employed for injections involving cords that impact the MCP joint compared to the PIP joint (0.39 mL versus 0.25 mL) resulting in a higher volume administered to the MCP joint than the PIP joint (0.31 mL versus 0.20 mL), while maintaining an equivalent total dose (0.58 mg). However, more than the maximum recommended dose of 0.25 mL of CCH has been demonstrated to be well tolerated and considered safe [28, 29].

By mixing 0.45 mL of diluent into the vial, this gives a constant dosing of 0.2 mg of Xiaflex® per 0.1 mL syringe gradation. Therefore, one can inject 0.1 mL (0.2 mg) three times, within 2–3 mm of each injection point, for essentially on-label dosing (0.60 vs 0.58 mg) [30]. Injection sites should be where the contracting cord is maximally separated from underlying tendons and skin is not adhered. Antiseptic is used and the patient's hand is secured for tension application. An assistant may be utilized to maintain this tension, so the injector has both hands available for injection [28]. Tension causes the cord to bowstring away from the joint and tendons.

The injector then exercises meticulous insertion of the needle, ensuring it does not pass entirely through the cord to avoid inadvertent injection into the surrounding tissue. If the needle is suspected to be in a tendon or the patient experiences paresthesia, the needle should be withdrawn and repositioned. Resistance during injection should be noted if the needle is in the proper location. The ideal circumstance is high resistance and slow flow of the injected fluid. Some recommend directing the needle obliquely through the cord, as opposed to in an anterior to posterior direction perpendicular to the hand, to avoid the flexor tendons [28].

Prudent, gradual injection is helpful to avert spillover of the enzyme into the subcutaneous tissues, where it is quickly metabolized by human proteases [30]. An aliquot of one-third of the solution is injected, and the needle is repositioned 2–3 mm both distal and proximal for full administration of the dose (Fig. 5.1). When cords are extremely thick, transverse alignment of the aliquots at one level may be useful for disruption. For a Y-cord that branches at the metacarpal head into adjacent fingers, injection at the branch point often corrects contracture in both digits [28].

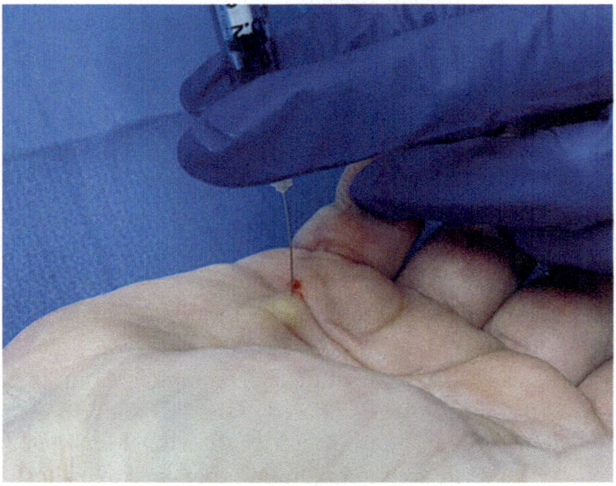

Fig. 5.1 Collagenase injections into Dupuytren's cord at 2 mm intervals

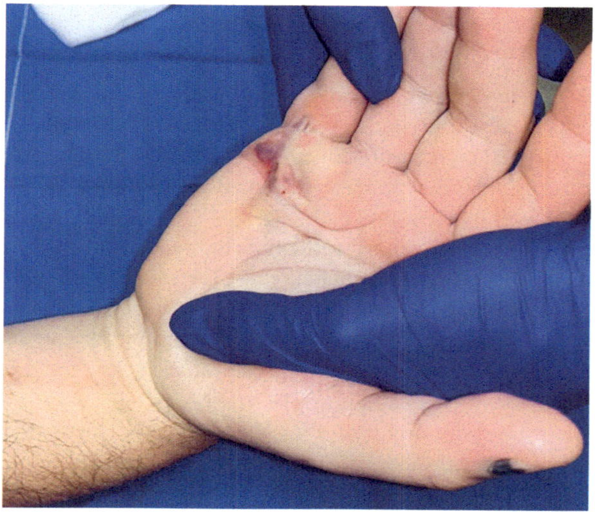

Fig. 5.2 Extension maneuver. Wrist in slight flexion, stabilize above and below involved joint and site of injection, steady pressure to extend the involved digit

When confronted with delivering dual injections on the same hand, initiation from an ulnar position and proceeding radially is the recommended course. In scenarios where both joints within a finger are impacted, the sequence commences proximally at the MCP joint and progresses distally to the PIP joint. After treatment, the patient's treated hand should be wrapped in a soft bulky dressing. Patients are advised to limit use, avoid self-manipulation to disrupt the injected cord(s), and keep extremity elevated [27].

Approximately 24–72 hours later, the manual finger extension procedure is performed to facilitate cord disruption if a contracture persists (Fig. 5.2). The extension maneuver should be performed in a proximal to distal fashion when both joints are injected in one digit. Local anesthesia may be used, and has in fact become standard of care, as research has shown improved correction with an anesthetic [31]. Care should be employed as some patients experience skin splitting, which should be treated with pressure for hemostasis and standard wound care dressings.

Manipulation has been performed up to 14 days post injection to allow for better control of skin splitting as swelling resolves [30]. With the patient's wrist flexed, controlled application of stretching pressure is applied to the injected cord by extending the finger for a period of 10–20 seconds. Cords involving the PIP joint should be extended with the MCP joint in a flexed position. A maximum of three attempts at finger extension may be performed at 5–10 minute intervals. If a cord fails to disrupt, a follow-up visit in 4 weeks should be scheduled, and if contraction persists, a supplementary treatment may be performed. Following finger extension, patients are instructed to perform finger flexion and extension exercises several times per day for several months. Additionally, it's advised to splint the digit in an extended position during nighttime hours [27].

5.2.1 Rehabilitation Protocol

At our institution, we only inject Xiaflex® into palmar cords. We have our patients return the following day for the extension maneuver. In our experience, patients with MCP contractures over 60 degrees are at higher risk for skin tearing (Fig. 5.3a, b). All patients who have sustained a tear had no long-term complications and did well with local wound care (Fig. 5.4a, b). Patients with less than 50 degrees of contracture can often have full extension restored with no adverse events (Figs. 5.5a, b and 5.6). We have the patients flex the involved finger after the cord breaks to confirm there was no tendon injury. After the cord disruption we send patients directly to Occupational Therapy (OT) for rehabilitation instructions and an extensor splint. OT recommends using a finger extensor splint for a full week, taking it off three times a day for gentle range of motion. After 1 week they then advise the patient to wear the splint nightly for another 4 weeks. This is dramatically less intensive than our recovery protocol after an open palmar fasciectomy where patients are instructed to wear the extensor splint full time for 1 month, with removal for range of motion three times a day, and then for another of 4 months of nightly splinting.

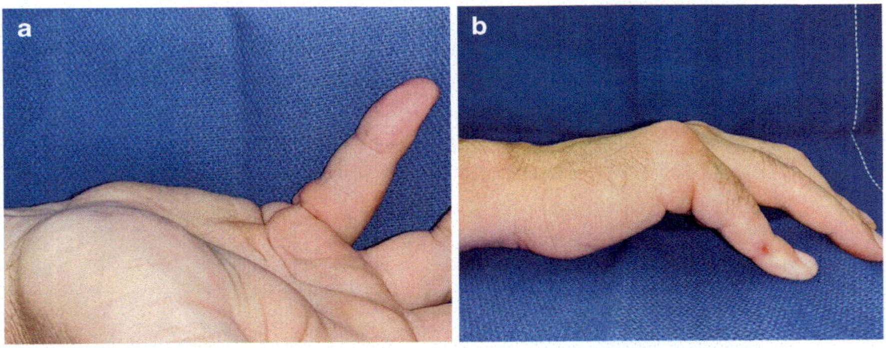

Fig. 5.3 Patient 1: Pre-collagenase injection. (**a**) At rest, small finger MCP contracture of 55°. (**b**) Trying to flatten hand against table

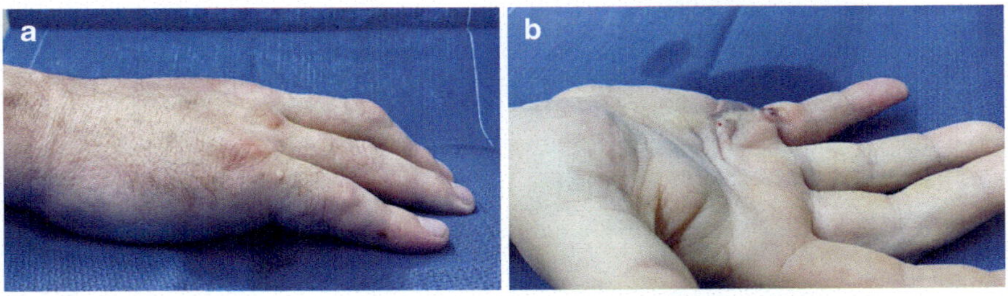

Fig. 5.4 Patient 1: Post-collagenase injection and manipulation. (**a**) Small finger MCP flexion of 10°. (**b**) Expected bruising, small skin tear at MCP joint

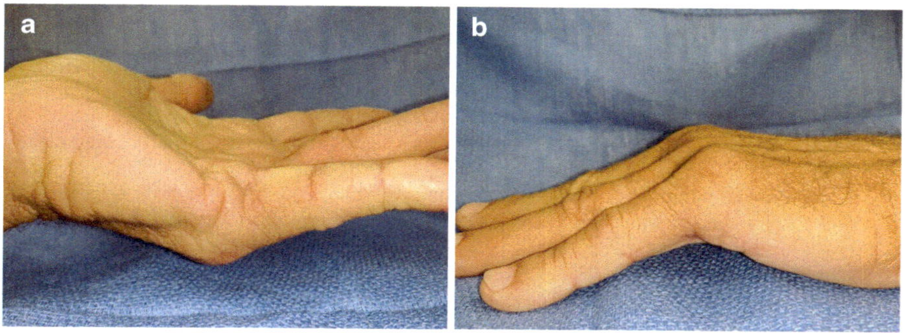

Fig. 5.5 Patient 2: Pre-collagenase injection. (**a**) At rest, small finger MCP contracture of 40°. (**b**) Trying to flatten hand against table

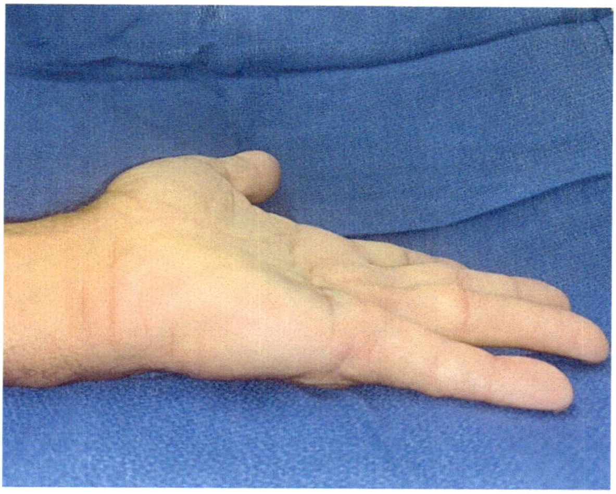

Fig. 5.6 Patient 2: Post-collagenase injection and manipulation with full small finger MCP extension

References

1. Kemler MA, de Wijn RS, van Rijssen AL, van Kooij YE, Ottenhoff M, et al. Dutch multidisciplinary guideline on Dupuytren disease. J Hand Surg Global Online. 2023;5:178–83. https://doi.org/10.1016/j.jhsg.2022.11.008.
2. Hurst LC, Badalamente MA, Hentz VR, Hotchkiss RN, Kaplan FT, Meals RA, Smith TM, Rodzvilla J. Injectable collagenase clostridium histolyticum for Dupuytren's contracture. N Engl J Med. 2009;361:968–79. https://doi.org/10.1056/NEJMoa0810866.
3. Thomas A, Bayat A. The emerging role of clostridium histolyticum collagenase in the treatment of Dupuytren disease. Ther Clin Risk Manag. 2010;6:557–72. https://doi.org/10.2147/TCRM.S8591.
4. Badalamente MA, Hurst LC. Efficacy and safety of injectable mixed collagenase subtypes in the treatment of Dupuytren's contracture. J Hand Surg Am. 2007;32(6):767–74. https://doi.org/10.1016/j.jhsa.2007.04.002.
5. Feldman G, Rozen N, Rubin G. Dupuytren's contracture: current treatment methods. IMAJ. 2017;19:648–50.

6. Warwick D, Arandes-Renú JM, Pajardi G, Witthaut J, Hurst LC. Collagenase clostridium histolyticum: emerging practice patterns and treatment advances. J Plast Surg Hand Surg. 2016;50:251–61. https://doi.org/10.3109/2000656X.2016.1159568.
7. Maclennan JD, Mandl I, Howes EL. Bacterial digestion of collagen. J Clin Invest. 1953;32:1317–22. https://doi.org/10.1172/JCI102860.
8. Hueston JT. Enzymic fasciotomy. Hand. 1971;3:38–40. https://doi.org/10.1016/0072-968x(71)90010-6.
9. Starkweather KD, Lattuga S, Hurst LC, Badalamente MA, Guilak F, Sampson SP, Dowd A, Wisch D. Collagenase in the treatment of Dupuytren's disease: an in vitro study. J Hand Surg Am. 1996;21:490–5. https://doi.org/10.1016/S0363-5023(96)80368-6.
10. Badalamente MA, Hurst LC. Enzyme injection as nonsurgical treatment of Dupuytren's disease. J Hand Surg Am. 2000;25:629–36. https://doi.org/10.1053/jhsu.2000.6918.
11. Badalamente MA, Hurst LC, Hentz VR. Collagen as a clinical target: nonoperative treatment of Dupuytren's disease. J Hand Surg Am. 2002;27:788–98. https://doi.org/10.1053/jhsu.2002.35299.
12. Badalamente MA, Hurst LC, Benhaim P, Cohen BM. Efficacy and safety of collagenase clostridium histolyticum in the treatment of proximal interphalangeal joints in dupuytren contracture: combined analysis of 4 phase 3 clinical trials. J Hand Surg Am. 2015;40:975–83. https://doi.org/10.1016/j.jhsa.2015.02.018.
13. Traore EJ, Wang W, Yafi FA, Hellstrom WJ. Collagenase clostridium histolyticum in the management of Peyronie's disease: a review of the evidence. Ther Adv Urol. 2016;8:192–202. https://doi.org/10.1177/1756287216637569.
14. Kang N, Sivakumar B, Sanders R, Nduka C, Gault D. Intra-lesional injections of collagenase are ineffective in the treatment of keloid and hypertrophic scars. J Plast Reconstr Aesthet Surg. 2006;59:693–9. https://doi.org/10.1016/j.bjps.2005.11.022.
15. Del Carlo M, Cole AA, Hart SGE, Levine LA. Comparative analysis of collagen degradation in Peyronie's disease plaque and Dupuytren's contracture cord tissues injected with mixed collagenase subtypes. J Urol. 2009;181:S279.
16. Xiaflex (clostridial collagenase histolyticum) Powder for Injection; 2010. https://www.accessdata.fda.gov/drugsatfda_docs/nda/2010/125338s000TOC.cfm. Accessed 4 Sep. 2023
17. Gilpin D, Coleman S, Hall S, Houston A, Karrasch J, Jones N. Injectable collagenase clostridium histolyticum: a new nonsurgical treatment for Dupuytren's disease. J Hand Surg Am. 2010;35:2027–38.e1. https://doi.org/10.1016/j.jhsa.2010.08.007.
18. Coleman S, Gilpin D, Kaplan FT, Houston A, Kaufman GJ, Cohen BM, Jones N, Tursi JP. Efficacy and safety of concurrent collagenase clostridium histolyticum injections for multiple Dupuytren contractures. J Hand Surg Am. 2014;39:57–64. https://doi.org/10.1016/j.jhsa.2013.10.002.
19. Peimer CA, Blazar P, Coleman S, Kaplan FT, Smith T, Lindau T. Dupuytren contracture recurrence following treatment with collagenase clostridium histolyticum (CORDLESS study): 3-year data. J Hand Surg Am. 2015;38(1):12–22.
20. Kan HJ, Verrijp FW, Hovius SE, van Nieuwenhoven CA, Selles RW. Recurrence of Dupuytren's contracture: a consensus-based definition. PLoS One. 2017;2017(12):e0164849. https://doi.org/10.1371/journal.pone.0164849.
21. Sahemey RS, Dhillon GS, Sagoo KS, Srinivas K. Cost-effectiveness and patient outcomes of injectable collagenase to treat Dupuytren's contracture. Cureus. 2021;13:e20530. https://doi.org/10.7759/cureus.20530.
22. Sefton AK, Smith BJ, Stewart DA. Cost comparison of collagenase clostridium histolyticum and fasciectomy for treatment of Dupuytren's contracture in the Australian health system. J Hand Surg (Asian-Pacific Volume). 2018;23:336–41. https://doi.org/10.1142/S2424835518500327.
23. Clesham K, Sheridan GA, Murphy EP, et al. Collagenase and the treatment of Dupuytren contracture: efficacy of treatment and patient satisfaction. J Hand Surg (Asian-Pacific Volume). 2022;27:141–7. https://doi.org/10.1142/S2424835522500138.

24. Bradley J, Warwick D. Patient satisfaction with collagenase. J Hand Surg Am. 2016;41:689–97. https://doi.org/10.1016/j.jhsa.2016.03.003.
25. Atroshi I, Nordenskjöld J, Lauritzson A, Ahlgren E, Waldau J, Walden M. Collagenase treatment of Dupuytren's contracture using a modified injection method: a prospective cohort study of skin tears in 164 hands, including short-term outcome. Acta Orthop. 2015;86:310–5. https://doi.org/10.3109/17453674.2015.1019782.
26. Grandizio LC, Akoon A, Heimbach J, Graham J, Klena JC. The use of residual collagenase for single digits with multiple-joint Dupuytren contractures. J Hand Surg Am. 2017;42:472.e1–6. https://doi.org/10.1016/j.jhsa.2017.03.001.
27. Endo Pharmaceuticals. Xiaflex (collagenase clostridium histolyticum) Prescribing Information. https://www.xiaflex.com/pdf/XIAFLEX_Prescribing_Information.pdf. Published August, 2022. Accessed 10 Sep 2023
28. Meals RA, Hentz VR. Technical tips for collagenase injection treatment for Dupuytren contracture. J Hand Surg Am. 2014;39:1195–200.e2. https://doi.org/10.1016/j.jhsa.2014.03.016.
29. Coleman S, Gilpin D, Tursi J, Kaufman G, Jones N, Cohen B. Multiple concurrent collagenase clostridium histolyticum injections to Dupuytren's cords: an exploratory study. BMC Musculoskelet Disord. 2012;13:61. https://doi.org/10.1186/1471-2474-13-61.
30. Murphy A, Lalonde DH, Eaton C, Denkler K, Hovius SER, Smith AA, Martin A, Biswas A, Van Nieuwenhoven C. Minimally invasive options in Dupuytren's contracture: aponeurotomy, enzymes, stretching, and fat grafting. Plast Reconstr Surg. 2014;134:822e–9e. https://doi.org/10.1097/PRS.0000000000000603.
31. Boe C, Blazar P, Iannuzzi N. Dupuytren contractures: an update of recent literature. J Hand Surg Am. 2021;46:896–906. https://doi.org/10.1016/j.jhsa.2021.07.005.

Chapter 6
Collagenase Injections: Evidence-Based Outcomes

Mark P. Smith and Reed Hoyer

Collagenase *Clostridium histolyticum* (CCH) was approved for use for Dupuytren's disease in the United States in 2010 by the FDA. Therefore, long-term follow-up of outcomes is limited. However, there is a growing body of evidence regarding its efficacy, safety, and outcomes that will be discussed in this chapter.

6.1 Phase II Trials

The efficacy and safety of CCH for Dupuytren's contractures has been studied and has been confirmed with multiple studies. In 2000, Badalamente and Hurst published early results of 35 patients with Dupuytren's disease in an open-label phase II trial. In their cohort, no major adverse reactions were experienced. An effective dose of 10,000 U was confirmed and early promising results were confirmed in patients who received this dose [1]. Following the confirmation of its safety and proposed efficacy, a series of randomized controlled trials (RCTs) sought to test the efficacy of CCH compared to placebo. In 2002, Badalamente et al. reported on a two-phase clinical study. In the first arm, the efficacy of 10,000 U of CCH versus a placebo injection was confirmed. In the second arm, 10,000 U was found to be the minimum safe and effective dose via a blinded study of various concentrations of CCH [2].

M. P. Smith
Department of Orthopaedic Surgery, Indiana University School of Medicine, Indianapolis, IN, USA
e-mail: maphsmit@iu.edu

R. Hoyer (✉)
Indiana Hand to Shoulder Center, Indianapolis, IN, USA
e-mail: rhoyer@ihtsc.com

M. B. Gottschalk et al. (eds.), *Dupuytren's Disease*,
https://doi.org/10.1007/978-3-031-85873-4_6

After the efficacy of CCH in Dupuytren's contractures was confirmed, Costas et al. sought to evaluate the efficacy of CCH in palmar Dupuytren's nodules. 75 patients with palpable nodules were enrolled in the RCT with a placebo control group. The size of the nodules was measured for a total of 8 weeks after the injection. The nodules decreased in size by 80% for 0.4 mg of CCH and 78% for 0.6 mg of CCH, which was statistically significant compared to placebo [3].

6.2 Phase III Trials

After phase II trials supported the efficacy of CCH for Dupuytren's contractures, the medication continued into phase III trials. Table 6.1 summarizes the clinical success rates of CCH from notable phase III trials. In 2007, Badalamente and Hurst performed a phase III trial of collagenase by enrolling 35 patients in a double-blinded placebo-controlled RCT. In the treatment group, 21 of 23 patients (91%) achieved a clinical success of reduction of contracture to less than five degrees, whereas 0% of the placebo group achieved clinical success. Up to three injections were performed as needed for treatment response. No severe adverse effects were experienced. Skin lacerations upon cord rupture were experienced in 11 patients, all of which were healed by secondary intention. The study was followed by an open-label extension, during which 35 joints were treated. Twenty-seven of 35 joints, or 77%, achieved clinical success during the open-label extension. Overall, an 87% clinical success rate was reported, requiring an average of 1.4 injections. A success rate of 90% was seen for MCP joints and 84% was seen for PIP joints. The patients were followed for 24 months. Of 62 joints injected, a recurrence was seen in four PIP joints and one MCP joint [4].

The Collagenase Option for Reduction of Dupuytren's (CORD) I Study Group in 2009 reported on a multi-center phase III placebo-controlled RCT of CCH in the treatment of Dupuytren's contractures. In their study, the CORD I Study Group evaluated 308 patients with fixed contractures of the metacarpophalangeal (MCP) or proximal interphalangeal (PIP) joints of over 20 degrees, excluding the thumb. The patients were followed for 30 days after their last injection. Patients were allowed to receive three injections of CCH, but more than half of the patients who failed CCH treatment did not receive all three injections. The CCH group

Table 6.1 Clinical success rate of CCH

Study	CCH clinical success rate (%)
Badalamente and Hurst [4]	77
Hurst et al. [5]	64
Gilpin et al. [6]	44
Peimer et al. [7]	65

Table of reported clinical success rate from phase III studies of all patients with Dupuytren's contractures treated with CCH. Clinical success is defined by the quoted study experienced improvement of contracture to less than five degrees in 64% of patients versus 6.8% in the placebo group. The CCH group experienced an average reduction in contracture from 50.2 to 12.2 degrees, whereas the placebo group experienced an average contracture reduction from 49.1 to 45.7 degrees. Upon further subanalysis, CCH achieved statistically significant reduction of contractures both of the MCP and PIP joints. The CCH group experienced a statistically significantly higher level of adverse effects from treatment. Ninety-six percent of the CCH cohort experienced an adverse effect from treatment, although most were mild. Severe adverse effects were experienced in the treatment group, three of which were treatment-related: one case of complex regional pain syndrome and two tendon ruptures. Overall, the authors concluded that CCH effectively reduces contractures and improves range of motion of the MCP and PIP joints secondary to Dupuytren's [5].

In 2010, the Collagenase Option for Reduction of Dupuytren's (CORD) II Study was published by Gilpin et al. The CORD II study took place in Australia, using a nearly identical protocol to the CORD I study. Sixty-four patients were followed for 90 days in this multi-center RCT. In their study, 44.4% of patients who received CCH achieved contractures less than five degrees compared to 4.8% of patients in the placebo group. Patients who received placebo experienced an average improvement in range of motion of 7.6 degrees, compared to 40 degrees in MCP joints treated with CCH and 32 degrees in PIP joints treated with CCH. One patient sustained a serious adverse event to CCH in their cohort: rapid proliferation of the Dupuytren's cord and a sensory abnormality [6].

6.3 Longer Follow-up of Case Series

The Collagenase Option for Reduction of Dupuytren Long-Term Evaluation of Safety Study (CORDLESS Study) was published in 2013, evaluating three-year recurrence rates after treatment of Dupuytren's with CCH. Patients from five previous studies who received at least one injection of CCH were enrolled in the CORDLESS study; a total of 643 patients were enrolled. Of 623 successfully treated joints, 65% of the joints revealed a sustained response to treatment with CCH. The recurrence rate for PIP joints was 56%, higher than that of MCP joints (27%). More of the successfully treated joints had low pretreatment severity versus high severity (79% versus 21%). Seven percent of successfully treated patients underwent medical or surgical management for Dupuytren's during the follow-up course. The authors note that the highest rate of recurrence was seen in patients with severe disease in the PIP joints. Adverse effects were seen in 193 of 643 patients, most of which were mild or moderate. Severe adverse effects were seen in 4.8% of patients, none of which were deemed to be directly related to the treatment with CCH [7].

In 2010, Watt et al. published eight-year outcomes of patients who received CCH for Dupuytren's. Patients who previously underwent phase II and III trials for CCH were contacted for long-term follow-up. Eight patients who underwent CCH treatment returned for eight-year follow-up, all treated with a single injection. Six patients were treated for MCP contractures, and two patients were treated for PIP contractures. No patients underwent further treatment. For patients with MCP contractures, the average contracture was 57 degrees before treatment, 9 degrees at 1 week, 11 degrees at 1 year, and 22 degrees at 8 years. For patients with PIP contractures, the average contracture was 40 degrees before treatment, 7.5 degrees at 1 week, 12.5 at 1 year, and 60 degrees at eight-year follow-up. Therefore, the patients with MCP contractures had much more durable results from CCH treatment than patients with PIP contractures [8].

6.4 Recurrent Collagenase Use

After the safety and efficacy of CCH was shown for the use of Dupuytren's, Bear et al. studied the efficacy of using CCH in recurrent contractures. Bear et al. published in 2016 on an open-label phase IV study in which 51 patients were treated for recurrent Dupuytren's contractures with recurrent injections of CCH. Patients who were treated in the CORDLESS study who experienced a recurrence of Dupuytren's contracture after treatment with CCH were eligible for inclusion in the study. For treatment of their recurrence, 69% of patients received one injection, 24% received two injections, and 8% received the maximum allotted three injections. The patients were followed clinically for 1 year after treatment. Of the patients treated, 57% achieved a contracture of less than five degrees. However, 67% of the patients who achieved a contracture of less than five degrees required three injections. Seventy-four percent of patients achieved an improvement in their range of motion of at least 20 degrees. In total, 86% of the patients achieved an improvement of range of motion of at least 20 degrees or achieved a contracture of less than five degrees. Forty-six of 52 patients experienced an adverse effect, with six reported severe adverse effects. No severe adverse reactions were determined to be treatment-related. Injection site pain was experienced in 19%, injection site swelling was experienced in 10%, and pruritis was experienced in 19% [9].

6.5 Concurrent Collagenase Use

Coleman et al. in 2014 sought to answer the question of whether CCH could safely and effectively be used for multiple joints in the same hand at the same time point. In this open-label, phase III study, 60 patients received two CCH injections into a single hand for two affected joints in one setting. Efficacy at 30 days post-treatment as well as adverse events were recorded. A 76% reduction in flexion contracture was reported. Three serious adverse events were experienced: one tendon rupture, one rupture of the A2-A4 pulleys, and one severe pain response. Therefore, the authors concluded that CCH is safe and effective in the short term for use of multiple concurrent joints [10].

In 2015, Gaston et al. published further data investigating the safety and efficacy of CCH in two joints concurrently. In a prospective study with 60-day follow-up, 715 patients underwent two concurrent injections for two joints of the same hand. The best improvement was seen in the two MCP joints subgroup with a 84% reduction in contracture and the lowest improvement was in the two PIP joints subgroup with a 60% reduction in contracture. Contracture of less than five degrees was seen in 65% of MCP joints and 29% of PIP joints. Six severe treatment-related adverse events occurred: one anaphylactic reaction, one tendon rupture, one hemorrhage, one case of lymphangitis, one incidence of deep venous thrombosis and pulmonary embolus, one patient with malaise, and one post-injection syncope of unknown origin. All adverse effects had similar rates compared to previous studies regarding one injection of CCH except skin lacerations. Twenty-two percent of the patients in this study experienced a skin laceration, which was higher than the published rates from a single injection ranging from 5% to 11%. Therefore, the authors concluded that concurrent use of CCH for two joints is equally as safe (except a higher risk of skin laceration) with similar efficacy to a single injection [11].

Cook et al. in 2019 published a retrospective cohort study comparing 117 patients who received a single injection of CCH to 59 patients who received more than one concurrent injection. A total of 121 joints were injected in the concurrent injection group. Over 80 percent of patients in both groups achieved immediate clinical success after their manipulation, and no difference between success rates was seen between the two cohorts. Adverse events were also evaluated. Lymphadenopathy was more common in the concurrent injection group, with a rate of 47.1% versus 28.8% for a single injection. However, no difference in the rate of adverse events otherwise was seen between the two cohorts [12].

6.6 Specific Considerations: Range of Disease Severity, Patient Characteristics

In 2018, Pess et al. published a *post-hoc* analysis of an open-label phase III study of CCH comparing the effect of CCH on different severities of Dupuytren's. In this open-label study, patients underwent two concurrent injections of CCH for two joint contractures of the same hand. The subanalysis reviewed 181 patients of various disease severities. No statistically significant differences were seen in treatment response to CCH based on disease severity. Additionally, the difference of treatment in MCP joints versus PIP joints was analyzed, with no significant difference seen [13].

Raven et al. in 2012 analyzed the effects of demographic information on the response to treatment with CCH. Patients from three previous RCTs were pooled. A total of 271 patients were included in the analysis. The patients were stratified by severity, sex, age, and diabetic status. No statistically significant differences in treatment response were seen in the different cohorts. No difference in the rate of adverse effects was seen between different subgroups [14].

6.7 Collagenase Versus Surgical Fasciectomy

Multiple studies have directly compared the treatment of CCH to surgical fasciectomy for treatment of Dupuytren's contractures. Table 6.2 summarizes the key findings in a select list of these comparative studies. In 2014, Atroshi et al. published a retrospective cohort study comparing short-term outcomes of CCH to that of surgical fasciectomy. Sixteen patients were treated with CCH and compared to 16 patients who underwent open fasciectomy. The patients were evaluated six weeks after treatment by a hand therapist. The median contracture of the CCH cohort and surgery cohort were both 10 degrees. Thus, in their study, the treatments had equivalent results in the short term [15].

Povlsen and Povlsen in 2014 also published their own review of patients who underwent CCH and surgical fasciectomy for single-digit contractures secondary to Dupuytren's. Ten patients were in each cohort. In their study, CCH had statistically significantly increased total range of motion as well as improved extension at the PIP joint, but surgery led to increased extension at the MCP joint compared to CCH [16].

Zhou et al. in 2015 sought to directly compare CCH to surgical fasciectomy for treatment of Dupuytren's. One hundred thirty-two patients were included in a matched cohort study. The authors found no statistically significant difference in the residual contractures after treatment with CCH versus surgical fasciectomy for MCP joints, with 13 degrees for CCH and six degrees for surgery. For PIP joints, CCH had worse residual contracture, with 25 degrees versus 15 degrees for surgery.

Table 6.2 Success rates of CCH compared to surgical fasciectomy

Study	Findings
Atroshi et al. [15]	Equivalent short-term results
Povlsen and Povlsen [6]	Surgery had better MCP extension
Zhou et al. [17]	CCH was equivalent for MCP joint but less effective for PIP joints. CCH had less adverse events and superior patient outcomes
Tay et al. [18]	Equivalent results, but surgery more effective for PIP
Leafblad et al. [19]	CCH had higher reintervention rate
Leclére et al. [20]	Equivalent for MCP joint. Surgery superior for PIP joint. CCH had superior patient satisfaction
Gruber et al. [21]	CCH had higher reintervention rate
Yamamoto et al. [22]	Equivalent patient outcome measures. CCH had higher recurrence

Table summarizing results of studies that compared CCH to surgical fasciectomy

Patient satisfaction scores were higher in the CCH group, and adverse events were less frequent for the CCH group. Therefore, the authors concluded that CCH was as effective as surgery for MCP joints, slightly less effective for PIP joints, but led to less adverse events and superior patient outcomes [17].

Tay et al. in 2015 retrospectively reviewed patients with Dupuytren's who were treated with CCH versus surgical fasciectomy. Thirty-seven patients were included in the study and were followed for at least 2 years. In their cohorts, partial fasciectomy led to less residual contracture than CCH for both MCP and PIP joints; partial fasciectomy led to contractures of 3.9 degrees for MCP joints and 6.5 degrees for PIP joints, and CCH led to contractures of 6.5 degrees for MCP joints and 40.6 degrees for PIP joints. The rate of complications was higher in the CCH group with a total of 26 complications versus 10 complications in the surgery cohort. All complications resolved without further treatment. No significant differences exist in patient satisfaction. Therefore, they concluded that both treatments are effective, but surgery may be more effective for contractures of the PIP joints [18].

Leafblad et al. performed a retrospective review comparing treatment of Dupuytren's with CCH to both surgical fasciectomy and needle aponeurotomy. Two hundred seventy-two treatments with CCH were performed and 132 open fasciectomies were performed. The two-year reintervention rate was 41% for CCH and 4% for open fasciectomy. The five-year reintervention rate was 55% for CCH and 4% for open fasciectomy. Younger age and severe PIP contracture were associated with increased risk of failure with CCH. Postintervention contracture measurements were not obtained in their study. Therefore, they concluded that CCH led to a higher reintervention rate than surgery [19].

In 2018, Leclére et al. performed a retrospective analysis of patients treated with CCH versus limited fasciectomy. Fifty-two patients were followed for 2 years. Surgical fasciectomy led to decreased contractures of PIP joints compared to CCH. Mean contractures for PIP joints for CCH were 51 degrees at baseline, 18 degrees at 6 weeks, and 32 degrees at 2 years. Mean contractures for PIP joints for surgery were 30 degrees at baseline, 2 degrees at 6 weeks, and 11 degrees at 2 years. Results were equivalent between groups for MCP joints. However, CCH led to increased patient satisfaction with 92% of patients stating they were satisfied with treatment compared to 71% in the surgery group. The CCH group had a 29% rate of minor complications [20].

Gruber et al. published a comparison between surgical fasciectomy and CCH for treatment of Dupuytren's in a single digit with longer-term follow-up. Telephone interviews with patients who underwent surgery or treatment with CCH were performed with at least a 5-year follow-up. Forty-four patients in each subgroup were included after propensity matching. At an average follow-up of 7.3 years, the CCH group had a higher rate of reintervention of 50% compared to 16% in the surgical fasciectomy group. Perceived disease recurrence was also higher in the CCH group, with 80% of patients experiencing recurrence versus 34% of the surgery cohort [21].

In 2022, Yamamoto et al. published a prospective non-randomized trial of parallel groups comparing CCH versus limited fasciectomy. Seventy-eight patients were analyzed. There was no difference in patient outcome measures for CCH compared to surgery. CCH showed a higher recurrence rate, at 18% versus 9.5%. No difference between residual contracture was seen for both MCP and PIP joints [22].

6.8 Collagenase Versus Percutaneous Needle Fasciotomy

CCH and percutaneous needle fasciotomy are two nonoperative treatment modalities that are utilized in the treatment of Dupuytren's contractures. Table 6.3 summarizes key findings from studies that compare these two treatment methods. In 2013, Nydick et al. directly compared the efficacy of CCH to percutaneous needle fasciotomy for Dupuytren's contractures. A retrospective review was performed comparing 29 patients treated with CCH and 30 patients treated with needle fasciotomy. The patients were followed for at least 3 months. Patient satisfaction was similar in the two groups, and no major complications were encountered in either group. Resolution of contracture to less than five degrees was seen in 67% of the needle fasciotomy group and 56% of the CCH group. Thus, the authors concluded that in the short term, the two treatments had similar success [23].

In 2016, Scherman et al. reported one-year results on an RCT regarding CCH versus needle fasciotomy. Ninety-six fingers were included in their analysis. No significant differences were seen in the residual contractures between groups at any time point, including the final time point at 1 year [24].

Skov et al. published an RCT in 2017 comparing CCH to percutaneous needle fasciotomy in patients with isolated PIP contractures secondary to Dupuytren's. Fifty patients were randomized and were followed for at least 2 years. Clinical success was defined as maintenance of contracture reduction less than 50% relative to baseline at two-year follow-up. Clinical success was seen in 7% of CCH patients and 29% of needle fasciotomy patients. The rate of complications was higher in the

Table 6.3 Success rates of CCH compared to needle fasciotomy

Study	Findings
Nydick et al. [23]	Similar success and patient outcomes
Scherman et al. [24]	Equivalent results
Skov et al. [25]	CCH had inferior outcomes with increased complication rate
Strömberg et al. [26]	Similar results
Strömberg et al. [27]	Similar results
Strömberg et al. [28]	Similar results
Leafblad et al. [19]	Similar reintervention rate
Abe [29]	Similar results
Jørgensen et al. [30]	CCH superior for MCP contractures
Byström et al. [31]	Similar results

Table summarizing results of studies that compared CCH to needle fasciotomy

CCH cohort, seen in 93% of patients versus 24% of patients in the CCH group, although most complications were transient and minor. They concluded that in their study, CCH had inferior outcomes to percutaneous needle fasciotomy for isolated PIP contractures [25].

In 2017, Strömberg et al. performed a study using ultrasound to evaluate the response after treatment with CCH versus percutaneous needle fasciotomy. Twenty patients underwent treatment with CCH and 19 patients underwent needle fasciotomy. No significant differences were observed between the cohorts with regard to the size of the rupture of the cord or in gain of mobility [26].

In 2018, Strömberg published two-year follow-up results of a randomized controlled study evaluating CCH versus needle fasciotomy. Seventy-six patients in each cohort completed the full two-year follow-up. Flexion contracture of less than five degrees was achieved in 88% of the CCH cohort and 90% of the needle fasciotomy of the cohort. The CCH cohort had increased rates of hematoma formation. The cohorts had a similar rate of skin ruptures, but the tears in the CCH group were larger. At one-year follow-up, no significant differences were observed between cohorts regarding contracture recurrence or patient outcomes [27]. At two-year follow-up, 76% of patients in the CCH group and 79% of the needle fasciotomy group maintained a contracture of less than five degrees. No differences were seen in patient-reported outcomes between the two cohorts [28].

In the previously discussed study by Leafblad et al., the CCH cohort was also compared to needle fasciotomy. There were 272 patients in the CCH group and 444 in the fasciotomy group. CCH had a 41% rate of reintervention at 2 years compared to 24% for needle fasciotomy. At 5 years, the two groups had a comparable rate of reintervention of 61% for needle fasciotomy and 55% for CCH [19].

In 2020, Abe published an RCT comparing clinical outcomes of CCH to needle fasciotomy. Seventy patients were randomized into the study and were followed for 3 years. All the MCP joints in both cohorts achieved a successful correction. Less severe PIP joint contractures achieved successful correction in 89% of the CCH patients and 100% of the needle fasciotomy group. Severe PIP contractures achieved successful correction in 50% of the CCH group and 67% of the needle fasciotomy group. Three-year recurrence for CCH was 26% for MCP joints, 44% for less severe PIP joints, and 67% for severe PIP joints. Three-year recurrence for needle fasciotomy was 29% of MCP joints, 38% of less severe PIP joints, and 67% of the severe PIP joints. Patient-reported outcomes at 30 days after treatment slightly favored needle fasciotomy. The authors concluded that both treatments are affective procedures for Dupuytren's with similar results. However, results are not as reliable for severe PIP contractures [29].

Jørgensen et al. in 2022 performed an RCT comparing rates of recurrence for patients treated with CCH versus percutaneous needle fasciotomy with three-year follow-up. Patients with isolated MCP contractures were included for the study. Thirty-six patients were randomized to receive needle fasciotomy and 32 patients received CCH. The rate of recurrence at 3 years was 47% for percutaneous needle fasciotomy compared to 19% for CCH, which was statistically significant. Therefore, the authors concluded that CCH was superior to needle fasciotomy for MCP contractures with regard to treatment efficacy and recurrence [30].

In 2022, Byström et al. published a prospective RCT with five-year follow-up comparing CCH and needle fasciotomy. One hundred fifty-six patients were divided evenly into the two groups. They found similar results between the groups. Extension deficits of less than five degrees were seen in 51% of the CCH group and 47% of the needle fasciotomy group. Recurrence rates were 56% for the CCH and 45% for the needle fasciotomy group [31].

6.9 Discussion

Collagenase *clostridium histolyticum* is a promising nonoperative modality to treat Dupuytren's contractures with a growing body of evidence since 2000. As a condition characterized by progressive proliferation of cords and progressive deformity, nonoperative treatment of Dupuytren's traditionally has been limited due to lack of efficacy and high rates of recurrence. However, CCH has shown successful short- and mid-term results, with a low rate of serious adverse effects. CCH is more successful for treatment of MCP joints than PIP joints. There is a high rate of minor adverse effects, with a low rate of severe adverse effects. When compared to surgical fasciectomy, CCH has similar efficacy, although it may be less effective for PIP joints. The recurrence rate is higher for CCH than surgery, although this may be an acceptable trade-off due to the less invasive nature of the treatment. When compared to percutaneous needle fasciotomy, CCH appears to be grossly equivalent with regards to efficacy and recurrence. Evidence exists to support CCH over needle fasciotomy, and vice versa. In conclusion, CCH appears to be an effective treatment for Dupuytren's contractures, especially of the MCP joint. Further studies are needed to compare outcomes of treatment options, but collagenase *Clostridium histolyticum* at this time is a useful option in the armamentarium of hand surgeons to treat Dupuytren's contractures.

References

1. Badalamente MA, Hurst LC. Enzyme injection as nonsurgical treatment of Dupuytren's disease. J Hand Surg Am. 2000;25(4):629–36. https://doi.org/10.1053/jhsu.200.
2. Badalamente MA, Hurst LC, Hentz VR. Collagen as a clinical target: nonoperative treatment of Dupuytren's disease. J Hand Surg Am. 2002;27(5):788–98. https://doi.org/10.1053/jhsu.2002.35299.
3. Costas B, Coleman S, Kaufman G, James R, Cohen B, Gaston RG. Efficacy and safety of collagenase Clostridium histolyticum for Dupuytren disease nodules: a randomized controlled trial. BMC Musculoskelet Disord. 2017;18(1):374.
4. Badalamente MA, Hurst LC. Efficacy and safety of injectable mixed collagenase subtypes in the treatment of Dupuytren's contracture. J Hand Surg Am. 2007;32(6):767–74. https://doi.org/10.1016/j.jhsa.2007.04.002.

5. Hurst LC, Badalamente MA, Hentz VR, et al. Injectable collagenase Clostridium histolyticum for Dupuytren's contracture. N Engl J Med. 2009;361(10):968–79. https://doi.org/10.1056/NEJMoa0810866.
6. Gilpin D, Coleman S, Hall S, Houston A, Karrasch J, Jones N. Injectable collagenase Clostridium histolyticum: a new nonsurgical treatment for Dupuytren's disease. J Hand Surg Am. 2010;35(12):2027–38.e1. https://doi.org/10.1016/j.jhsa.2010.08.007.
7. Peimer CA, Blazar P, Coleman S, et al. Dupuytren contracture recurrence following treatment with collagenase Clostridium histolyticum (CORD LESS study): 3-year data. J Hand Surg Am. 2013;38(1):12–22. https://doi.org/10.1016/j.jhsa.2012.09.028.
8. Watt AJ, Curtin CM, Hentz VR. Collagenase injection as nonsurgical treatment of Dupuytren's disease: 8-year follow-up. J Hand Surg Am. 2010;35(4):534–539.e1. https://doi.org/10.1016/j.jhsa.2010.01.003.
9. Bear BJ, Peimer CA, Kaplan FTD, Kaufman GJ, Tursi JP, Smith T. Treatment of recurrent dupuytren contracture in joints previously effectively treated with collagenase Clostridium histolyticum. J Hand Surg Am. 2017;42(5):391.e1–8. https://doi.org/10.1016/j.jhsa.2017.02.010.
10. Coleman S, Gilpin D, Kaplan FT, et al. Efficacy and safety of concurrent collagenase Clostridium histolyticum injections for multiple Dupuytren contractures. J Hand Surg Am. 2014;39(1):57–64. https://doi.org/10.1016/j.jhsa.2013.10.002.
11. Gaston RG, Larsen SE, Pess GM, et al. The efficacy and safety of concurrent collagenase Clostridium histolyticum injections for 2 Dupuytren contractures in the same hand: a prospective, multicenter study. J Hand Surg Am. 2015;40(10):1963–71. https://doi.org/10.1016/j.jhsa.2015.06.099.
12. Cook J, Waughtel J, Andreoni AR, Sakharpe A, Friedman DW. Collagenase Clostridium histolyticum for Dupuytren's contracture: comparing single and concurrent injections. Plast Reconstr Surg. 2019;143(4):782e–7e. https://doi.org/10.1097/PRS.0000000000005443.
13. Pess GM, Sundbom M, Wilson K, Lindqvist D, Dahlin LB. A *post hoc* analysis of Dupuytren contracture treated with collagenase *Clostridium histolyticum* across disease stages. J Plast Surg Hand Surg. 2018;52(5):301–6. https://doi.org/10.1080/2000656X.2018.1484753.
14. Raven RB 3rd, Kushner H, Nguyen D, Naam N, Curtin C. Analysis of efficacy and safety of treatment with collagenase Clostridium histolyticum among subgroups of patients with Dupuytren contracture. Ann Plast Surg. 2014;73(3):286–90. https://doi.org/10.1097/SAP.0b013e31827ae9d0.
15. Atroshi I, Strandberg E, Lauritzson A, Ahlgren E, Waldén M. Costs for collagenase injections compared with fasciectomy in the treatment of Dupuytren's contracture: a retrospective cohort study. BMJ Open. 2014;4(1):e004166.
16. Povlsen B, Povlsen SD. What is the better treatment for single digit dupuytren's contracture: surgical release or collagenase clostridium histolyticum (Xiapex) injection? Hand Surg. 2014;19(3):389–92. https://doi.org/10.1142/S0218810414500324.
17. Zhou C, Hovius SER, Slijper HP, et al. Collagenase clostridium histolyticum versus limited fasciectomy for Dupuytren's contracture: outcomes from a multicenter propensity score matched study. Plast Reconstr Surg. 2015;136(1):87–97. https://doi.org/10.1097/PRS.0000000000001320.
18. Tay TK, Tien H, Lim EY. Comparison between collagenase injection and partial fasciectomy in the treatment of Dupuytren's contracture. Hand Surg. 2015;20(3):386–90. https://doi.org/10.1142/S0218810415500288.
19. Leafblad ND, Wagner E, Wanderman NR, et al. Outcomes and direct costs of needle aponeurotomy, collagenase injection, and fasciectomy in the treatment of Dupuytren contracture. J Hand Surg Am. 2019;44(11):919–27. https://doi.org/10.1016/j.jhsa.2019.07.017.
20. Leclère FM, Kohl S, Varonier C, Unglaub F, Vögelin E. Range of motion, postoperative rehabilitation and patient satisfaction in MCP and PIP joints affected by Dupuytren Tubiana stage 1-3: collagenase enzymatic fasciotomy or limited fasciectomy? A clinical study in 52 patients. Arch Orthop Trauma Surg. 2018;138(11):1623–31. https://doi.org/10.1007/s00402-018-3034-6.

21. Gruber JS, Zhang D, Janssen SJ, Blazar P, Jupiter JB, Earp BE. Limited fasciectomy versus collagenase clostridium histolyticum for dupuytren contracture: a propensity score matched study of single digit treatment with minimum 5 years of telephone follow-up. J Hand Surg Am. 2021;46(10):888–95. https://doi.org/10.1016/j.jhsa.2021.05.022.
22. Yamamoto M, Yasunaga H, Kakinoki R, et al. The CeCORD-J study on collagenase injection versus aponeurectomy for Dupuytren's contracture compared by hand function and cost effectiveness. Sci Rep. 2022;12(1):9094.
23. Nydick JA, Olliff BW, Garcia MJ, Hess AV, Stone JD. A comparison of percutaneous needle fasciotomy and collagenase injection for dupuytren disease. J Hand Surg Am. 2013;38(12):2377–80. https://doi.org/10.1016/j.jhsa.2013.08.096.
24. Scherman P, Jenmalm P, Dahlin LB. Three-year recurrence of Dupuytren's contracture after needle fasciotomy and collagenase injection: a two-centre randomized controlled trial. J Hand Surg Eur. 2018;43(8):836–40. https://doi.org/10.1177/1753193418786947.
25. Skov ST, Bisgaard T, Søndergaard P, Lange J. Injectable collagenase versus percutaneous needle fasciotomy for Dupuytren contracture in proximal interphalangeal joints: a randomized controlled trial. J Hand Surg Am. 2017;42(5):321–328.e3. https://doi.org/10.1016/j.jhsa.2017.03.003.
26. Strömberg J, Vanek P, Fridén J, Aurell Y. Ultrasonographic examination of the ruptured cord after collagenase treatment or needle fasciotomy for Dupuytren's contracture. J Hand Surg Eur. 2017;42(7):683–8. https://doi.org/10.1177/1753193417711594.
27. Strömberg J, Ibsen-Sörensen A, Fridén J. Comparison of treatment outcome after collagenase and needle fasciotomy for Dupuytren contracture: a randomized, single-blinded, clinical trial with a 1-year follow-up. J Hand Surg Am. 2016;41(9):873–80. https://doi.org/10.1016/j.jhsa.2016.06.014.
28. Strömberg J, Ibsen Sörensen A, Fridén J. Percutaneous needle fasciotomy versus collagenase treatment for Dupuytren contracture: a randomized controlled trial with a two-year follow-up. J Bone Joint Surg Am. 2018;100(13):1079–86. https://doi.org/10.2106/JBJS.17.01128.
29. Abe Y. Comparison of treatment outcomes after collagenase injection and percutaneous needle fasciotomy for Dupuytren's contracture: objective and subjective comparisons with a 3-year follow-up. Plast Reconstr Surg. 2020;145(6):1464–74. https://doi.org/10.1097/PRS.0000000000006828.
30. Jørgensen RW, Jensen CH, Jørring S. Three-year recurrence of Dupuytren contracture after needle fasciotomy or collagenase injection: a randomized controlled trial. Plast Reconstr Surg. 2023;151(2):365–71. https://doi.org/10.1097/PRS.0000000000009847.
31. Byström M, Ibsen Sörensen A, Samuelsson K, Fridén JO, Strömberg J. Five-year results of a randomized, controlled trial of collagenase treatment compared with needle fasciotomy for Dupuytren contracture. J Hand Surg Am. 2022;47(3):211–7. https://doi.org/10.1016/j.jhsa.2021.11.019.

Chapter 7
Open Fasciectomy: Background and Techniques

Kitty Y. Wu and Marco Rizzo

7.1 Indications

While Dupuytren's disease is typically painless, progressive contractures can lead to ongoing functional limitation. The Hueston tabletop test, considered positive when patients are unable to place their hands flat on a tabletop, is often used as a threshold for consideration of treatment intervention [1] (Fig. 7.1). Patients are often indicated for surgery if they have greater than 30° metacarpophalangeal (MCP) flexion contracture or any degree of proximal interphalangeal (PIP) joint contracture, skin breakdown or matted disease, or recurrent disease resulting in limitations in hand function. Patients with Dupuytren's diathesis have features suggestive of a more aggressive disease course, including bilateral disease, ectopic lesions outside of the palm (Garrod's knuckle pads, Lederhose's disease, Peyronie's disease), strong family history, male gender, and age of onset younger than 50 years [2]. These patients have an increased risk of recurrence of 71% compared to the baseline risk of 23% and may be indicated for surgical intervention earlier.

7.2 Anesthesia

Open fasciectomy can be performed under local anesthesia, regional block with sedation, or general anesthesia depending on disease severity and patient and surgeon comfort level. A recent Canadian study comparing WALANT (wide-awake local anesthetic no tourniquet) to general anesthesia with a tourniquet demonstrated similar range of motion outcomes following fasciectomy [3]. Further considerations

K. Y. Wu · M. Rizzo (✉)
Department of Orthopedic Surgery, Mayo Clinic, Rochester, MN, USA
e-mail: Rizzo.Marco@mayo.edu

M. B. Gottschalk et al. (eds.), *Dupuytren's Disease*,
https://doi.org/10.1007/978-3-031-85873-4_7

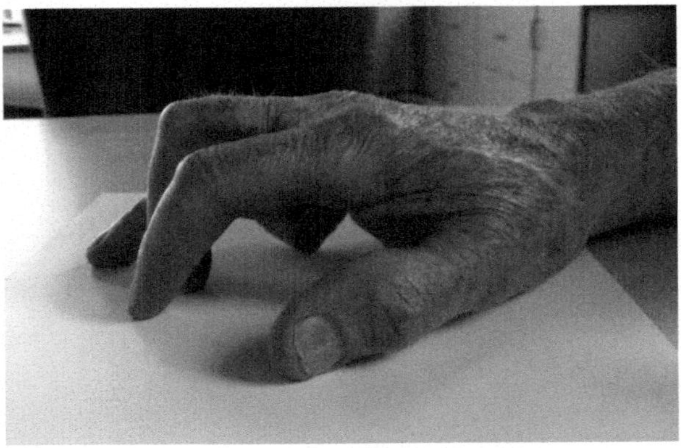

Fig. 7.1 Hueston tabletop test. A positive tabletop test, where the patient is unable to place their hand flat on tabletop, is often used as an indication for surgical intervention for Dupuytren's contracture

include whether full-thickness skin grafting is required and donor site location, as well as recurrent disease that may present a more challenging dissection.

If the procedure is being performed under wide-awake local anesthesia, lidocaine with 1:100000 epinephrine is commonly used for analgesia. Use of a 30-gauge needle and buffering with sodium bicarbonate can help decrease the pain of injection. Waiting at least 30 minutes after injection prior to starting the procedure to allow for the epinephrine to reach maximal vasoconstriction [4]. In a review of 203 consecutive cases of Dupuytren's fasciectomy performed with epinephrine, there were no ischemic digital complications; however, this technique is contraindicated in patients with true allergy to local anesthetic medications and significant peripheral vascular disease including Buerger's disease, Raynaud's, scleroderma, vasculitis, and sickle cell anemia [3, 5, 6].

7.3 Surgical Options

Surgical options include fasciotomy (transection of the diseased cord without excision); local fasciectomy (conservative excision of involved fascia); regional fasciectomy (more extensive excision of involved fascia); radical/total fasciectomy (removal of all diseased palmar fascia); open palm McCash technique (transverse palm incision allowing healing by secondary intention); and dermatofasciectomy (excision of involved skin and fascia). The choice of technique should be individualized to the patient, taking into consideration disease severity, medical comorbidities, required recovery time, and ability to perform dressing changes and engage in hand therapy.

7.3.1 Fasciotomy

Surgical fasciotomy, similar to percutaneous needle aponeurotomy, involves transection and release of the thickened cords with a scalpel. This can be performed under local anesthesia through limited incisions directly overlying the cords and is associated with relatively fast post-operative recovery. This procedure may be well-suited for patients who are elderly, with low functional demands or medical comorbidities that may not be able to tolerate a longer procedure, or those at high risk for wound healing issues. This technique may also be used in conjunction with the application of a skeletal extension torque frame (Chap. 9).

7.3.2 Fasciectomy

A local, regional, or radical fasciectomy involves excision of the diseased thickened palmar fascia to varying extents. Various skin flaps can be utilized including Bruner incisions, midline longitudinal incision with multiple Z-plasties, or a combination of both (Chap. 12) (Fig. 7.2).

After skin incision, skin flaps should be elevated and kept as thick as possible to avoid flap necrosis. Within the palm, flaps can be safely elevated with a blade above the level of the palmar fascia. In areas where the diseased fascia is close to or

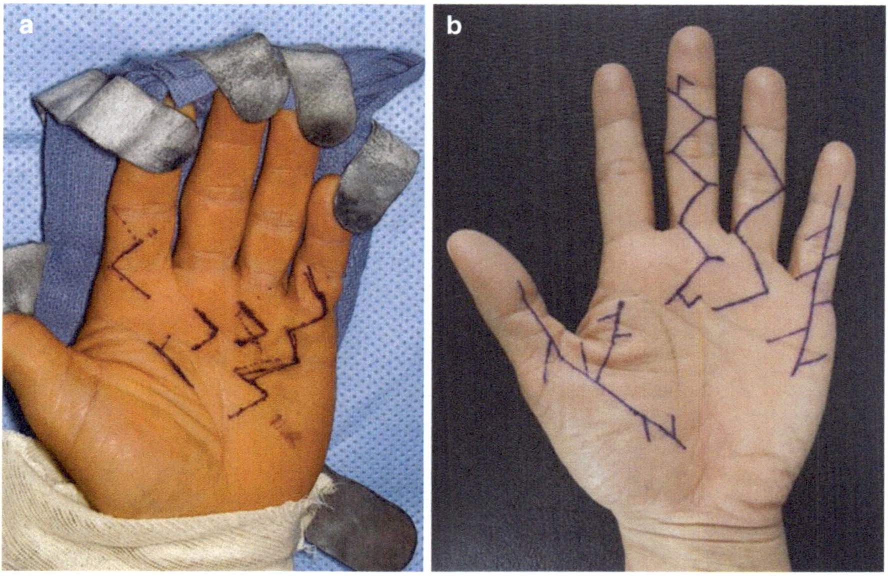

Fig. 7.2 Fasciectomy incisions. (**a**) Bruner type incisions and (**b**) midline longitudinal incisions with Z-plasties (thumb and small finger) can be used

involves the dermis, care should be taken to avoid causing "button-holes" within the skin flaps. One method is to color the palmar skin using a purple marking pen in these areas. When raising the flap, if the color starts to become visible on the deep surface of the skin flap as it is being raised, this should raise caution that the flap is becoming too thin. The radial and ulnar neurovascular bundle on either side of the cord should be identified proximally within the palm and then followed distally into the digit (Fig. 7.3a). Dissection should be performed with care and microsurgical instruments, if needed, to avoid neurapraxic injury to the digital nerves. Spiral cords within the digit cause superficial and midline displacement of the digital nerves, so care should be taken to ensure they are fully visualized prior to the excision of any diseased cords (Fig. 7.4). Similarly, within the webspaces, the common digital nerve bifurcating into the two digital nerves should be clearly visualized prior to cord excision (Fig. 7.3b). The cord can then be transected proximally and then dissected from the underlying flexor tendon sheath using a blade. At this step, care should be taken to preserve the flexor tendon sheath and underlying pulleys. The neurovascular bundle can be gently retracted medially to excise any retrovascular disease which is most often the cause of distal interphalangeal joint contractures. Some authors advocate for the excision of the diseased fascia with 3-5 mm margins and inclusion of the vertical septae of Legueu and Juvara as a means of reducing recurrence rates [7]. Firm gentle pressure can then be used to passively extend the digit.

If there is residual PIP joint contracture following excision of the diseased palmar fascia, then a step-wise approach can be utilized to address other potential causative structures limiting full extension [8]. First, the A3 pulley and any taut cruciate bands are released. If a flexion contracture persists, the transverse retinacular ligament is then divided followed by a checkrein ligament release. Next, a PIP joint capsulotomy and collateral ligament release is performed and lastly a volar plate release. If there is still recalcitrant PIP joint contracture then either acceptance of the deformity or PIP joint arthrodesis can be considered.

If a tourniquet is used, this should always be let down prior to skin closure and meticulous hemostasis should be obtained. The skin incision can then be closed

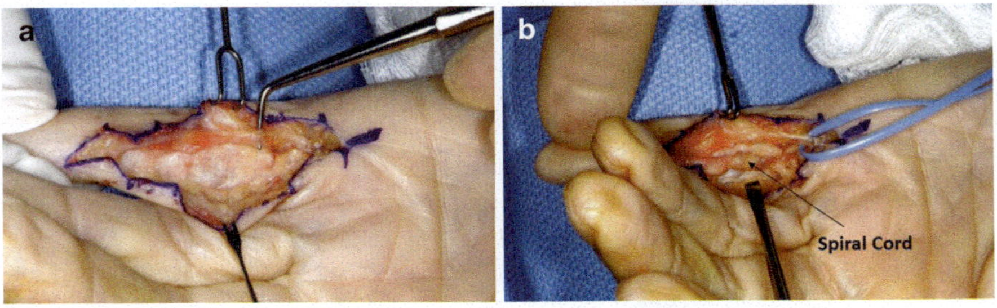

Fig. 7.3 Neurovascular bundle dissection. (**a**) After raising of the skin flaps, the radial digital nerve is dissected from proximal to distal (green microsurgical background). (**b**) The common digital nerve bifurcating into the proper digital nerves must be visualized and protected within the webspace prior to excision of the diseased palmar fascia

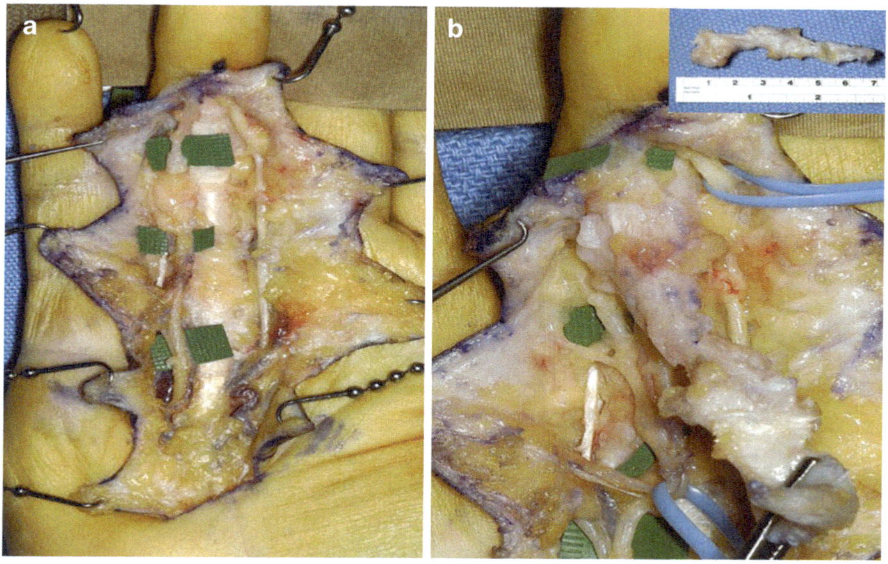

Fig. 7.4 Spiral Dupuytren's cord. (**a**) The spiral cord results displace the ulnar digital nerve (probe) medially and superficially. (**b**) Once digital nerve is identified (blue vessel loop) the spiral cord can be isolated for excision

primarily or with Z-plasties. Full-thickness skin grafting may be required in cases of severe contractures and can be harvested from the ipsilateral medial forearm, hypothenar area, or upper arm.

7.3.3 McCash Open Palm Technique

McCash described this technique to address MP joint flexion contractures by utilizing a transverse incision within the distal palmar crease and leaving this incision to heal by secondary intention with the patient placed in an extension splint [9]. The advantages of this technique include a lower risk of skin necrosis and hematoma formation, limited dissection resulting in decreased post-operative stiffness, and minimal reported pain [10]. Disadvantages, however, include the poor visualization of neurovascular structures, risk of infection, need for daily dressing and wound care, and patient concerns regarding unsightly cosmesis with an open wound.

Lesiak et al. described a modification of the McCash technique involving the similar use of a transverse incision with the addition of a full-thickness skin graft to hasten healing and avoid prolonged period of time with open wounds [10].

7.3.4 Dermatofasciectomy and Full-Thickness Skin Grafting

First described by Hueston in 1962 for patients with Dupuytren's diathesis or recurrent disease, dermatofasciectomy involves the entire excision of the thickened cords and overlying skin, followed by coverage with a full-thickness skin graft [11, 12]. The skin excision extends from the palmar digital crease to the proximal or distal interphalangeal joint crease and encompasses the entirety of the volar skin between the mid-axial lines. A full-thickness skin graft can be harvested from the ipsilateral medial forearm or upper arm to provide coverage over the exposed flexor tendon and neurovascular bundles.

7.4 Post-operative Care

Following local, regional, or radical fasciectomy, patients are placed in a forearm-based volar resting splint and early range of motion is encouraged within a week post-operatively. Patients undergoing the McCash open palm release or dermatofasciectomy can start range of motion as soon as pain allows and skin graft healing is ensured. Nighttime splinting is continued until 6 weeks post-operative.

7.5 Complications

Complications following treatment include post-operative hematoma, delayed wound healing or skin flap necrosis, flexor tendon injury, digital nerve neurapraxia or transection, and digital arterial injury. Post-operative hematomas can lead to skin flap compromise and necrosis and should be decompressed in the office setting or evacuated in the operating room in a timely fashion. Resulting areas of skin flap necrosis can be managed conservatively with dressing changes and allowed to heal by secondary intention. Suspected flexor tendon or digital nerve injuries should be addressed immediately with operative exploration and repair as necessary. One of the most feared complications is digital arterial injury resulting in a dysvascular digit. Arterial vasospasm can often lead to the appearance of a dysvascular digit after tourniquet release. Intraoperative measures including flexion of the digit to relieve any undue tension, re-warming the digit, and application of papaverine or lidocaine should be implemented. If an adverse reaction to epinephrine is suspected, reversal with phentolamine injection should be administered [13]. If there is persistent ischemia and inadequate return of capillary refill, then exploration and revascularization procedures should be considered.

7.6 Conclusions

The surgical management of Dupuytren's contracture involves a variety of techniques ranging from limited fasciotomy to extensive resection of both the skin and underlying diseased cords. As Dupuytren's disease is not curable, recurrence is part of the expected natural history with enough time. The decision for surgical intervention should be shared between the patient and surgeon balancing the potential of faster disease recurrence with the invasiveness of the procedure.

References

1. Hueston JT. The table top test. Hand. 1982;14(1):100–3. https://doi.org/10.1016/s0072-968x(82)80053-3.
2. Hindocha S, Stanley JK, Watson S, Bayat A. Dupuytren's diathesis revisited: evaluation of prognostic indicators for risk of disease recurrence. J Hand Surg Am. 2006;31(10):1626–34. https://doi.org/10.1016/j.jhsa.2006.09.006.
3. Nelson R, Higgins A, Conrad J, Bell M, Lalonde D. The wide-awake approach to Dupuytren's disease: fasciectomy under local anesthetic with epinephrine. Hand. 2010;5(2):117–24. https://doi.org/10.1007/s11552-009-9239-y.
4. McKee DE, Lalonde DH, Thoma A, Dickson L. Achieving the optimal epinephrine effect in wide awake hand surgery using local anesthesia without a tourniquet. Hand. 2015;10(4):613–5. https://doi.org/10.1007/s11552-015-9759-6.
5. Barone N, Lalonde DH, Brutus JP. Tips, tricks, and pearls for a superior patient and surgeon experience for wide-awake Dupuytren surgery. Plast Reconstr Surg Glob Open. 2024;12(2):e5570. https://doi.org/10.1097/GOX.0000000000005570.
6. Lalonde D, Bell M, Benoit P, Sparkes G, Denkler K, Chang P. A multicenter prospective study of 3,110 consecutive cases of elective epinephrine use in the fingers and hand: the Dalhousie project clinical phase. J Hand Surg Am. 2005;30(5):1061–7. https://doi.org/10.1016/j.jhsa.2005.05.006.
7. Miranda BH, Elliott C, Kearsey CC, et al. 3-dimensional fasciectomy: a highly efficacious common ground approach to Dupuytren's surgery. Arch Plast Surg. 2018;45(6):557–63. https://doi.org/10.5999/aps.2016.02131.
8. Denkler KA, Park KM, Alser O. Treatment options for Dupuytren's disease: tips and tricks. Plast Reconstr Surg Glob Open. 2022;10(1):e4046. https://doi.org/10.1097/GOX.0000000000004046.
9. McCash CR. The open palm technique in Dupuytren's contracture. Br J Plast Surg. 1964;17:271–80. https://doi.org/10.1016/s0007-1226(64)80043-6.
10. Lesiak AC, Jarrett NJ, Imbriglia JE. Modified McCash technique for management of Dupuytren contracture. J Hand Surg Am. 2017;42(5):395. https://doi.org/10.1016/j.jhsa.2017.01.018.
11. Hueston JT. Recurrent Dupuytren's contracture. Plast Reconstr Surg. 1963;31:66–9. https://doi.org/10.1097/00006534-196301000-00008.
12. Hueston JT. Digital Wolfe grafts in recurrent Dupuytren's contracture. Plast Reconstr Surg Transplant Bull. 1962;29:342–4. https://doi.org/10.1097/00006534-196204000-00005.
13. Aljahany MS, Aleid DK, Aal Ibrahim AM. Reversal of digital ischemia with Phentolamine after accidental epinephrine injection. Am J Case Rep. 2020;21:e923877. https://doi.org/10.12659/AJCR.923877.

Chapter 8
Open Fasciectomy: Evidence-Based Outcomes

Eric Mitchell and Joshua Gillis

8.1 Introduction

Open fasciectomy techniques for Dupuytren's disease broadly include limited, radical, and dermo-fasciectomy. Studies examining radical and dermo-fasciectomy technique outcomes are generally more historical and less prevalent given they have fallen out of favour with most surgeons. The outcomes of these techniques will be discussed later in this chapter, while the outcomes for limited fasciectomy are outlined below.

8.2 Early Operative Outcomes

Significant improvement in total extension deficits is seen early in the post-operative course at the one-week mark, with an average 73% reduction in deficits across all joints seen. Average improvement at the MCP was from 42° to 9° on average (83% improvement), and from 34° to 14° at the PIPJ (53% improvement) [1]. Further improvement can be seen between one and 6 weeks as the healing process continues and largely ceases by this time. The six-week point should serve as a new baseline for patients having undergone open fasciectomy in terms of total range of motion improvement [1].

E. Mitchell
Division of Plastic Surgery, Western University, London, ON, Canada

J. Gillis (✉)
Division of Plastic Surgery, NL Health Services, Memorial University, St. John's, NL, Canada
e-mail: js964286@dal.ca

M. B. Gottschalk et al. (eds.), *Dupuytren's Disease*,
https://doi.org/10.1007/978-3-031-85873-4_8

Some amount of residual deformity is expected after open limited fasciectomy, particularly for the PIP joint, even despite additional joint release intra-operatively. Residual contracture at the MCP averages from 0° to –9° at early follow-up and greater residual deformity is seen at the PIP, averaging 9–14° [1–3]. Overall improvement in contracture correction occurs in the MCP joint as compared to the PIP, with average improvement of 80–95% and 44–53%, respectively [1–3]. Zhou et al. evaluated the early outcomes at an average of 10 weeks in 215 patients who underwent limited fasciectomy [3]. They found total residual extension deficits across the MCP and PIP joints decreased 71% from 61° to 18°. Another study of 36 fingers undergoing limited fasciectomy found total residual extension deficits across both joints decreased from 67.8° to 15.9° post-op at 6 weeks. This included MCP contracture decreasing from 35.3° to 1.7°, and PIP joint contracture decreasing from 32.5° to 14.3° [2].

8.3 Residual PIPJ Contracture Management

In order to achieve maximal intra-operative improvement in PIP joint contracture and minimize residual deformity after surgery, multiple techniques have been described. Additional PIP joint release is often required in those with severe deformity [4, 5]. Gentle passive manipulation can be done first after baseline fasciectomy is complete and also should be done after any additional joint release [6]. If, after completion of the fasciectomy intra-operatively, further contracture remains (>20–25°), release of the volar check rein ligaments is recommended, followed by release of the accessory collateral ligaments, and then entire volar plate [7]. Incision of the flexor tendon sheath at the level of the A3 pulley may be another means of improving PIP join correction [8].

Hohendroff et al. examined the impact of supplementary arthrolysis at the PIP joint intra-operatively for 16 digits with primary Dupuytren's disease [9]. Median PIP flexion contracture was 84° pre-operatively and 30° post-op, despite complete extension being possible at the PIP joint intra-operatively in 94% of cases digits. Weinzweig et al. conducted a retrospective review of 42 PIP joints with 60° or greater contracture [10]. Fasciectomy alone was performed in 27 joints and 15 joints underwent fasciectomy and capsulotomy. Mean improvement in contracture was 53% in the non-capsulotomy group (78.4° pre-op to 36.6° post-op), compared to 55% in the capsulotomy group (82.5° pre-op to 36.8° post-op) at average follow-up of 10 and 6 months, respectively. Intra-operative residual contracture was 7° for the non-capsulotomy group and 8° for the capsulotomy group. Ritchie et al. found fasciectomy alone improved PIP joint flexion contracture in eight digits from 28° to 1° immediately post-op, 6° at 3 months, and 8° at 36 months [4]. Eleven digits underwent fasciectomy and sequential PIP joint release. Mean pre-operative flexion contracture was 70°, which improved to 42° after fasciectomy, and 7° of residual deformity after joint release, immediately post-op. Three-month contracture was 26° and 29° at 36 months. This study suggests the long-term residual deformity in the PIP joint for severe contractures is better after supplementary joint release, compared to fasciectomy alone [4].

Several studies have examined the impact of releasing specific peri-articular structures in cases of PIP joint contracture from Dupuytren's disease. One study recommends making a transverse incision at the A3 pulley of the flexor tendon sheath for cases of residual intra-operative PIP joint contracture [8]. In 22 joints, mean pre-operative PIP joint contracture was 58°, which improved to 28° after fasciectomy alone, and subsequent release of the flexor tendon sheath improved mean contracture to 5°. Eight digits had a mean residual contracture of 13°. A study by Watson et al. achieved full intra-operative extension in 110 out of 115 PIP joints with any amount of flexion contracture from various causes including Dupuytren's disease, after release of the checkrein ligaments alone [7]. Another study found fasciectomy alone improved PIP joint contracture from 78° pre-operatively to 62° after fasciectomy, and subsequent capsuloligamentous release further improved average joint contracture to 2° intra-operatively [11]. Average contracture at 6 months was 16°. In this study, incising the flexor tendon sheath at the distal end of the A2 pulley alone did not correct the PIP joint contracture in any patients.

A study by Trickett et al. suggested residual intra-operative contracture at the PIP joint may be secondary to under-resected retrovascular cords [5]. 99 consecutive digits in 73 patients were included, with a mean pre-operative flexion contracture at the PIP joint of 69°. Excision of the central cord alone improved PIP joint contracture by 44%. Excision of the spiral or lateral cords, and retrovascular cords improved contractures by 19% and 23%, respectively. In cases where PIP joint contracture was still >25°, the accessory collateral ligaments were released. Not all types of cords were present in all digits that were operated on, but this study highlights the importance of structures such as the retrovascular cords. The importance of the retrovascular cord was also identified by McFarlane as a cause of under-corrected PIP joint deformity [12].

8.4 Late Operative Outcomes

The early improvement seen in degree of joint contracture tends to be stable over time in the majority of patients. Significant improvements are seen many years out, with complete and sustained correction of MCP contracture in 70% of patients [13, 14]. At 12 months, 87% of patients have what is considered to be a functional level of range of motion of at least 165° [14]. Similar to differences between joints at early follow-up, complete correction long-term at the PIP joint is less common [13].

Average joint contracture multiple years after open fasciectomy ranges from 6° to 20° at the PIPJ compared to 0–11° at the MCP [15–19]. Wei et al. [20] evaluated the outcomes of open partial fasciectomy in 19 patients at a minimum of 2-year follow-up. Pre-operative passive extension deficits of the MCP and PIP joints were 44.8° and 50.7°, respectively. At the final follow-up, MCP and PIP joint extension deficits were 3.9 (reduction of 91%) and 6.5 (reduction of 87%) degrees, respectively. At an average of 39 months post-operatively, another study of 21 patients undergoing limited fasciectomy found MCP joint contracture decreased from 41.4° pre-operatively to 3.7 post-operatively, and PIP contractures decreased from 29.9 to 8.1 post-operatively [17].

Patient satisfaction after open fasciectomy is high, with 71–92% of patients satisfied with their results at 2–5 years, which is similar to contracture improvement in that it remains stable over time [16–19].

8.4.1 Self-reported Recovery of Hand Function

A majority of patients considered their hand function to be much better or fully recovered after limited fasciectomy by 6 months post-operative, with no further improvement of self-reported recovery after that time-point [14]. Patient-reported outcome scores have found a similar significant improvement in function compared to pre-operatively that persists over time [15, 16, 21, 22].

8.5 Recurrence

Recurrence of contracture after fasciectomy has been reported in multiple ways in the literature. A consensus definition of recurrence developed in 2017 stated it as *"an increase in joint contracture in any treated joint of at least 20° at one-year post-treatment compared to six weeks post-treatment"* [23]. Not all reports of recurrence in the literature have used this consensus definition.

Studies using the consensus definition have found an average recurrence rate of 3–39% at 5 years after limited fasciectomy [19, 24, 25]. Another study found a 20% recurrence rate at an average of 7 years post-operatively [26]. When recurrence occurs, it is usually within the first few years after surgery [27]. Not all patients who develop a recurrence require re-intervention, with re-intervention rates after primary open fasciectomy ranging from 0% to 7% at 5 years [15, 28, 29].

The rate of extension or progression of disease is a separate entity from recurrence and refers to contracture progression outside of the immediate site of previous surgery. The rate of extension after open fasciectomy is generally higher than that of recurrence [30].

8.6 Predictors of Outcomes

In patients undergoing open fasciectomy there are some factors that may affect outcomes. In general, more mild contractures achieve greater absolute improvement in range of motion, compared to more severe contractures [2, 31]. As a result, we recommend counselling patients using expected per cent improvement in contracture, rather than providing an absolute prediction in number of degrees.

As previously mentioned, the PIP joint achieves worse outcomes as compared to the MCP in terms of residual deformity and per cent improvement in contracture. This may be related to anatomical differences in the joints. A flexed MCP joint as a result of Dupuytren's disease is in an anatomical position, whereas the anatomic position of the PIP joint is in extension. Prolonged flexion at the PIP joint results in shortening and contracture of the soft tissues around the joint, i.e., the collateral ligaments, volar plate and intrinsic musculature. This difference explains why additional joint release is often required for severe PIP joint contractures, and why even dividing the collateral ligaments and volar plate may not be sufficient to achieve complete correction of joint position.

Operating on multiple digits in a single procedure may have a negative impact on the amount of absolute improvement gained in range of motion [27]; however, studies are conflicting [14]. Recurrence rate has not been found to be associated with number of digits operated on [27]. Scarring does tend to be worse, likely related to multiple incisions and an overall higher burden for post-operative healing. Inherent density or volume of disease is often greater in these cases which may also present a more aggressive form of Dupuytren's.

Age at the time of surgery is another factor of interest. Higher age at the time of surgery may predict lower recurrence rate [19]; however, younger age at the time of surgery has been associated with more functional improvement (i.e., DASH scores) compared to older patients [32]. A study of patient-reported outcomes in 54 patients who underwent limited fasciectomy found a correlation between patient age and functional improvement (DASH score) at 12 months post-op, with younger patients reporting larger improvement compared to older patients. This could relate to higher functional demands of younger individuals.

The presence of Dupuytren's diathesis features has been thought of as predicting more aggressive and recurrent disease [33]; however, this has not been borne out consistently in the literature [19]. Specific features of Dupuytren's diathesis, like radial digits having contracture, do have worse outcomes compared to ulnar digits [34].

Post-operative splinting has not been found to have a significant effect on outcomes after open fasciectomy. A randomized-control trial found no significant differences between patients who received a static night-time extension splint plus therapy for 6 months compared to therapy alone, in 154 patients who underwent either dermo-fasciectomy or limited fasciectomy [35]. A systematic review and meta-analysis of four randomized-control trials found no difference between patients receiving a post-operative splint compared to those who do not on total extension deficits at 3 months or patient-reported outcomes [36]. Although not supported by existing literature, some recommend continuing with splint therapy at the 2-week post-operative mark if there is a net loss of extension that has occurred at that point [35, 36].

8.7 Complications

The overall complication rate after limited fasciectomy ranges from 10%–25% for mild complications and 1–2% for serious complications [3, 24, 37, 38]. Complications can be categorized based on timing—peri-operative, early post-operative, and late post-operative.

Peri-operative complications typically involve injury to the neurovascular bundle, with reported rates of 3–6% and 0–5% to nerves and arteries, respectively [15, 24, 38–40].

If digital ischemia is appreciated intra-operatively, surgeons should consider loosening compression from sutures, the dressing, or by decreasing the amount of finger extension. Infiltration of agents such as papaverine or plain lidocaine without epinephrine can be considered as well. If there is no improvement in the vascular status of the digit at that point, or if injury to either structure was visualized intra-operatively, exploration and potential micro-surgical repair is recommended.

Early post-operative complications are generally mild, with the most common concerns being wound healing or flap necrosis, infection, and transient neuropraxia. Wound healing or flap necrosis generally improves with ongoing dressing care and rarely requires additional intervention. The rate of this complication is around 2–10% [15, 24, 27, 30, 38, 40]. Infection occurs at a rate of 0–12% [2, 13, 29, 30, 37–39].

Neuropraxia at a rate of 0–52% [30, 37, 39, 40]. Hematomas are less common at 2% of cases [38–40]. Stiffness and flexion deficits are to be expected after fasciectomy, and thankfully often temporary. We recommend range of motion be initiated as soon as 2–3 days post-operatively with direction from registered hand therapists, particularly in older patients. This can be in conjunction with a nighttime resting orthosis, if deemed necessary.

Late complications are most commonly complex regional pain syndrome (CRPS) or ongoing sensory disturbance. CRPS can be very debilitating, and it is reported as occurring in 0–10% of cases [24, 29, 30, 38, 40]. Recurrence can be considered a late complication as well, with the typical outcomes previously described previously in this chapter.

8.8 Other Open Fasciectomy Techniques and Outcomes

The outcomes of radical fasciectomy were examined by McIndoe and Beare [41]. This study deemed results as generally “satisfactory” in a series of over 200 patients and highlighted their impression that better results occurred in patients during earlier stages of Dupuytren’s disease. Another study from 1967 evaluated 122 patients who underwent radical fasciectomy for 153 hands, with a follow-up range of one to 15 years, and found a recurrence rate of 22% and disease extension rate of 21% [42]. A comparison of limited versus radical fasciectomy late-term results between

5 and 15 years found no significant differences in recurrence, extension, or secondary surgery rates [43]. Roulet et al. examined the long-term results of "extensive" fasciectomy combined with the McCash open technique [27]. At 7 years post-op, there was a 17% recurrence rate, and 37% rate of disease extension, with 90% of patients deeming their result to be "good". Flexion contracture improved from 39° at the MCP, and 32 at the PIP pre-operatively, to 2° at the MCP and 15° at the PIP.

There are some studies that have evaluated the outcomes of dermo-fasciectomy and also comparing dermo-fasciectomy to limited fasciectomy. One study reported no recurrence of diseased tissue, but an 8% extension rate, in 36 hands treated with dermo-fasciectomy at an average 3.9-year follow-up [44]. Recurrence was found to be 11.6% in another study of 103 patients at an average follow-up of 5.8 years [45]. Two-point discrimination has been reported at a mean of 8 mm for the digits at 8 years post DF [46].

When comparing the outcomes of limited fasciectomy and dermo-fasciectomy, Rodrigues et al. found a 0% re-operation rate for DF at 1 and 5 years post-operative, compared to 2.5% and 7.1% for LF, respectively [29]. However, the rate of "poor" outcomes was 58.5% in DF compared to LF. Rates of infection and cold intolerance at follow-up were also higher in DF patients compared to LF (14.9% versus 8.8% for infection, 29.4% versus 15.9% for cold sensitivity at 5 years). Tonkin et al. also compared DF to LF in 100 patients, finding 54% recurrence in the fasciectomy group compared to 33–42% in the grafting groups [47]. Improvement in total extension lag was 52% in DF patients and 58% in LF patients. Time return to work and activity were also greater in DF patients compared to fasciectomy. Dermo-fasciectomy has historically been recommended for more extensive and aggressive Dupuytren's disease.

References

1. van Rijssen AL, Gerbrandy FSJ, Ter Linden H, Klip H, Werker PMN. A comparison of the direct outcomes of percutaneous needle fasciotomy and limited fasciectomy for Dupuytren's disease: a 6-week follow-up study. J Hand Surg. 2006;31:717–25. https://doi.org/10.1016/j.jhsa.2006.02.021.
2. Noureddine H, Vejsbjerg K, Harrop JE, White MJ, Chakravarthy J, Harrison JWK. Fasciectomy under local anaesthetic and adrenaline for Dupuytren's contracture in a community setting in the UK with a cost analysis. Bone Joint J. 2020;102:1354–8. https://doi.org/10.1302/0301-620X.102B10.BJJ-2019-1685.R2.
3. Zhou C, Selles RW, Slijper HP, Feitz R, van Kooij Y, Moojen TM, Hovius SER. Comparative Effectiveness of percutaneous needle aponeurotomy and limited fasciectomy for Dupuytren's contracture: a multicenter observational study. Plast Reconstr Surg. 2016;138:837–46. https://doi.org/10.1097/PRS.0000000000002560.
4. Ritchie JFS, Venu KM, Pillai K, Yanni DH. Proximal interphalangeal joint release in Dupuytren's disease of the little finger. J Hand. 2004;29:15–7. https://doi.org/10.1016/j.jhsb.2003.08.005.
5. Trickett RW, Savage R, Logan AJ. Angular correction related to excision of specific cords in fasciectomy for Dupuytren's disease. J Hand Surg. 2014;39:472–6. https://doi.org/10.1177/1753193413502161.

6. Breed CM, Smith PJ. A comparison of methods of treatment of pip joint contractures in Dupuytren's disease. J Hand Surg. 1996;21:246–51. https://doi.org/10.1016/s0266-7681(96)80107-0.
7. Watson HK, Light TR, Johnson TR. Checkrein resection for flexion contracture of the middle joint. J Hand Surg. 1979;4:67–71. https://doi.org/10.1016/s0363-5023(79)80107-0.
8. Blazar PE, Floyd EW, Earp BE. The quantitative role of flexor sheath incision in correcting Dupuytren proximal interphalangeal joint contractures. J Hand Surg. 2016;41:609–13. https://doi.org/10.1177/1753193415602189.
9. Hohendorff B, Spies CK, Müller LP, Ries C. Supplementary arthrolysis of the proximal interphalangeal finger joint in Dupuytren's contracture: primary operation versus revision. Arch Orthop Trauma Surg. 2016;136:435–9. https://doi.org/10.1007/s00402-015-2380-x.
10. Weinzweig N, Culver JE, Fleegler EJ. Severe contractures of the proximal interphalangeal joint in Dupuytren's disease: combined fasciectomy with capsuloligamentous release versus fasciectomy alone. Plast Reconstr Surg. 1996;97:560–6.; discussion 567. https://doi.org/10.1097/00006534-199603000-00011.
11. Beyermann K, Prommersberger KJ, Jacobs C, Lanz UB. Severe contracture of the proximal interphalangeal joint in Dupuytren's disease: does capsuloligamentous release improve outcome? J Hand Surg. 2004;29:240–3. https://doi.org/10.1016/j.jhsb.2004.02.002.
12. McFarlane RM. The current status of Dupuytren's disease. J Hand Surg. 1983;8:703–8. https://doi.org/10.1016/s0363-5023(83)80251-2.
13. Eckerdal D, Lauritzson A, Nordenskjöld J, Åkesson A, Atroshi I. Finger joint contractures 5 years after treatment for Dupuytren disease: a comparative cohort study of collagenase injection versus surgical fasciectomy. J Hand Surg. 2022;47:834–42. https://doi.org/10.1016/j.jhsa.2022.04.019.
14. Engstrand C, Krevers B, Nylander G, Kvist J. Hand function and quality of life before and after fasciectomy for Dupuytren contracture. J Hand Surg. 2014;39:1333–1343.e2. https://doi.org/10.1016/j.jhsa.2014.04.029.
15. Bergovec M, Jelicic J, Oljaca A, Bilic R. Hand function and recurrence after limited fasciectomy for Dupuytren's contracture: long-term follow-up. J Orthop Surg Hong Kong. 2018;26:2309499018762195. https://doi.org/10.1177/2309499018762195.
16. Leclère FM, Kohl S, Varonier C, Unglaub F, Vögelin E. Range of motion, postoperative rehabilitation and patient satisfaction in MCP and PIP joints affected by Dupuytren Tubiana stage 1-3: collagenase enzymatic fasciotomy or limited fasciectomy? A clinical study in 52 patients. Arch Orthop Trauma Surg. 2018;138:1623–31. https://doi.org/10.1007/s00402-018-3034-6.
17. Naam NH. Functional outcome of collagenase injections compared with fasciectomy in treatment of Dupuytren's contracture. Hand. 2013;8:410–6. https://doi.org/10.1007/s11552-013-9540-7.
18. Tay TKW, Tien H, Lim EYL. Comparison between collagenase injection and partial fasciectomy in the treatment of Dupuytren's contracture. Hand Surg. 2015;20:386–90. https://doi.org/10.1142/S0218810415500288.
19. van Rijssen AL, Ter Linden H, Werker PMN. Five-year results of a randomized clinical trial on treatment in Dupuytren's disease: percutaneous needle fasciotomy versus limited fasciectomy. Plast Reconstr Surg. 2012;129:469–77. https://doi.org/10.1097/PRS.0b013e31823aea95.
20. Tay TK, Tien H, Lim EY. Comparison between Collagenase Injection and Partial Fasciectomy in the Treatment of Dupuytren's Contracture. Hand surgery: an international journal devoted to hand and upper limb surgery and related research: journal of the Asia-Pacific Federation of Societies for Surgery of the Hand. 2015;20(3):386–90. https://doi.org/10.1142/S0218810415500288.
21. Kitridis D, Karamitsou P, Giannaros I, Papadakis N, Sinopidis C, Givissis P. Dupuytren's disease: limited fasciectomy, night splinting, and hand exercises-long-term results. Eur J Orthop Surg Traumatol. 2019;29:349–55. https://doi.org/10.1007/s00590-018-2340-6.

22. Thoma A, Kaur MN, Ignacy TA, Levis C, Martin S, Duku E, Haines T. Health-related quality of life in patients undergoing palmar fasciectomy for Dupuytren's disease. Plast Reconstr Surg. 2014;133:1411–9. https://doi.org/10.1097/PRS.0000000000000177.
23. Kan HJ, Verrijp FW, Hovius SER, van Nieuwenhoven CA, Dupuytren Delphi Group, Selles RW. Recurrence of Dupuytren's contracture: a consensus-based definition. PLoS One. 2017;12:e0164849. https://doi.org/10.1371/journal.pone.0164849.
24. Radhamony NG, Nair RR, Sreenivasan S, Walkay S, Soni A, Kakkar R. Residual deformity versus recurrence following Dupuytren's palmar fasciectomy-a long term follow-up of 142 cases. Ann Med Surg. 2022;2012(73):103224. https://doi.org/10.1016/j.amsu.2021.103224.
25. Selles RW, Zhou C, Kan HJ, Wouters RM, van Nieuwenhoven CA, Hovius SER. Percutaneous aponeurotomy and lipofilling versus limited fasciectomy for Dupuytren's contracture: 5-year results from a randomized clinical trial. Plast Reconstr Surg. 2018;142:1523–31. https://doi.org/10.1097/PRS.0000000000004982.
26. Mavrogenis AF, Spyridonos SG, Ignatiadis IA, Antonopoulos D, Papagelopoulos PJ. Partial fasciectomy for Dupuytren's contractures. J Surg Orthop Adv. 2009;18:106–10.
27. Roulet S, Bacle G, Guéry J, Charruau B, Marteau E, Laulan J. Outcomes at 7 and 21 years after surgical treatment of Dupuytren's disease by fasciectomy and open-palm technique. Hand Surg Rehabil. 2018;37:305–10. https://doi.org/10.1016/j.hansur.2018.05.007.
28. Leafblad ND, Wagner E, Wanderman NR, Anderson GR, Visscher SL, Maradit Kremers H, Larson DR, Rizzo M. Outcomes and direct costs of needle aponeurotomy, collagenase injection, and fasciectomy in the treatment of Dupuytren contracture. J Hand Surg. 2019;44:919–27. https://doi.org/10.1016/j.jhsa.2019.07.017.
29. Rodrigues JN, Zhang W, Scammell BE, Chakrabarti I, Russell PG, Fullilove S, Davidson D, Davis TRC. Functional outcome and complications following surgery for Dupuytren's disease: a multi-centre cross-sectional study. J Hand Surg Eur. 2017;42:7–17. https://doi.org/10.1177/1753193416660045.
30. Chen NC, Srinivasan RC, Shauver MJ, Chung KC. A systematic review of outcomes of fasciotomy, aponeurotomy, and collagenase treatments for Dupuytren's contracture. Hand. 2011;6:250–5. https://doi.org/10.1007/s11552-011-9326-8.
31. Stepić N, Končar J, Rajović M. The influence of Dupuytren's disease fingers contracture degree on surgical treatment outcome. Vojnosanit Pregl. 2017;74:19–23. https://doi.org/10.2298/VSP150331103S.
32. Zyluk A, Jagielski W. The effect of the severity of the Dupuytren's contracture on the function of the hand before and after surgery. J Hand Surg. 2007;32:326–9. https://doi.org/10.1016/J.JHSB.2006.10.007.
33. Abe Y, Rokkaku T, Ofuchi S, Tokunaga S, Takahashi K, Moriya H. An objective method to evaluate the risk of recurrence and extension of Dupuytren's disease. J. Hand Surg. 2004a;29:427–30. https://doi.org/10.1016/j.jhsb.2004.06.004.
34. Abe Y, Rokkaku T, Ofuchi S, Tokunaga S, Takahashi K, Moriya H. Dupuytren's disease on the radial aspect of the hand: report on 135 hands in Japanese patients. J Hand Surg Edinb Scotl. 2004b;29:359–62. https://doi.org/10.1016/j.jhsb.2003.12.007.
35. Jerosch-Herold C, Shepstone L, Chojnowski AJ, Larson D, Barrett E, Vaughan SP. Night-time splinting after fasciectomy or dermo-fasciectomy for Dupuytren's contracture: a pragmatic, multi-centre, randomised controlled trial. BMC Musculoskelet Disord. 2011;12:136. https://doi.org/10.1186/1471-2474-12-136.
36. Karam M, Kahlar N, Abul A, Rahman S, Pinder R. Comparison of hand therapy with or without splinting postfasciectomy for Dupuytren's contracture: systematic review and meta-analysis. J Hand Microsurg. 2021;14:308–14. https://doi.org/10.1055/s-0041-1725221.
37. Bulstrode NW, Jemec B, Smith PJ. The complications of Dupuytren's contracture surgery. J Hand Surg. 2005;30:1021–5. https://doi.org/10.1016/j.jhsa.2005.05.008.
38. Krefter C, Marks M, Hensler S, Herren DB, Calcagni M. Complications after treating Dupuytren's disease. A systematic literature review. Hand Surg Rehabil. 2017;36:322–9. https://doi.org/10.1016/j.hansur.2017.07.002.

39. Denkler K. Surgical complications associated with fasciectomy for Dupuytren's disease: a 20-year review of the English literature. Eplasty. 2010;10:e15.
40. Peimer CA, Wilbrand S, Gerber RA, Chapman D, Szczypa PP. Safety and tolerability of collagenase Clostridium histolyticum and fasciectomy for Dupuytren's contracture. J Hand Surg. 2015;40:141–9. https://doi.org/10.1177/1753193414528843.
41. McINDOE A, Beare RL. The surgical management of Dupuytren's contracture. Am J Surg. 1958;95:197–203. https://doi.org/10.1016/0002-9610(58)90502-6.
42. Dickie WR, Hughes NC. Dupuytren's contracture: a review of the late results of radical fasciectomy. Br J Plast Surg. 1967;20:311–4. https://doi.org/10.1016/s0007-1226(67)80055-9.
43. Hueston JT. Limited fasciectomy for Dupuytren's contracture. Plast Reconstr Surg Transplant Bull. 1961;27:569–85. https://doi.org/10.1097/00006534-196106000-00001.
44. Ketchum LD, Hixson FP. Dermofasciectomy and full-thickness grafts in the treatment of Dupuytren's contracture. J Hand Surg. 1987;12:659–63. https://doi.org/10.1016/S0363-5023(87)80043-6.
45. Armstrong JR, Hurren JS, Logan AM. Dermofasciectomy in the management of Dupuytren's disease. J Bone Joint Surg Br. 2000;82:90–4. https://doi.org/10.1302/0301-620x.82b1.9808.
46. Brotherston TM, Balakrishnan C, Milner RH, Brown HG. Long term follow-up of dermofasciectomy for Dupuytren's contracture. Br J Plast Surg. 1994;47:440–3. https://doi.org/10.1016/0007-1226(94)90075-2.
47. Tonkin MA, Burke FD, Varian JP. Dupuytren's contracture: a comparative study of fasciectomy and dermofasciectomy in one hundred patients. J Hand Surg. 1984;9:156–62.

Chapter 9
Continuous Extension Torque: Background, Technique, and Evidence-Based Outcomes

Adil Shahzad Ahmed

9.1 Background

Severe cases of Dupuytren's contracture significantly impair patient function. The flexed finger posture blocks the ability of the hand to grasp and manipulate objects. Traditional surgical fasciectomy in these cases is challenging due to limited anatomic space when the finger is closed in the palm, and there is elevated risk of neurovascular injury secondary to restricted visualization [1, 2]. Severe cases can further experience subpar outcomes from incomplete resection given the above limitations and risks. Additionally, acute complete correction in severe contracture may lead to finger ischemia and possible necrosis from the sudden stretch placed on chronically shortened digital vessels [3].

Staged management in these settings can be advantageous. This was traditionally performed via splinting, casting, and stretching techniques, aiming to permanently elongate the tissue via synthesis of new collagen [4, 5]. However, these methods did not provide complete correction and often led to dorsal skin ulceration, ischemia, and necrosis [6]. More recent techniques have evolved, utilizing external fixation to achieve similar correction [7, 8]. Via initial application of an external fixator, gradual and progressive correction of a contracture can be accomplished. This is frequently followed in the second stage by fixator removal and traditional open fasciectomy.

There are many different external fixation devices, some designed specifically for Dupuytren's contracture correction while others have more diverse uses. Examples include the Agee Digit Widget (Hand Biomechanics Lab, Inc., Sacramento, California), Tecnica di Estensione Continua (TEC) [9], Verona [10], PIPSTER (Proximal Interphalangeal Skeletal Traction Extender) [11], Multiplanar

A. S. Ahmed (✉)
Joseph Barnhart Department of Orthopaedic Surgery, Baylor College of Medicine, Houston, TX, USA

M. B. Gottschalk et al. (eds.), *Dupuytren's Disease*,
https://doi.org/10.1007/978-3-031-85873-4_9

[12], Compass Hinge [13], S-Quattro [14], and traditional Ilizarov-type external fixation [8]. Despite the design and instrumentation differences, the underlying principle in these and other devices is gradual correction of the flexion contracture via extension torque applied through bony fixation.

9.2 Technique

Given the variety of external fixation options as listed above, there is no single "universal" surgical technique. Each device has its own specific methodology, based on the position and number of pins, guide-assisted versus freehand placement, uniplane versus multi-plane fixation, and hand-based orthosis for correction versus intra-frame mechanism for correction. More relevant than detailing stepwise techniques for each device are the general indications and considerations for use.

Staged treatment with initial continuous extension torque can be considered for Dupuytren's contracture cases with proximal interphalangeal (PIP) joint flexion contractures. Not every PIP joint flexion contracture requires preliminary external fixation-assisted extension prior to surgery, and there are no concrete guidelines regarding exact flexion contracture values, as different ranges are reported [15–17]. Some authors posit that PIP flexion contractures greater than 30° can be considered severe and thought should be given to preliminary application of external extension torque [15]. This is ultimately dictated by surgeon preference and comfort, and open discussion with the patient regarding relative merits, timeframe of expected treatment, potential complications, and willingness or ability to participate in treatment. Concomitant flexion contracture at the metacarpophalangeal (MCP) joint is common in severe cases, such as when the finger is curled into the palm. Although these devices were traditionally developed to target and treat PIP joint flexion contractures, they may be able to successfully address concomitant flexion contractures at the MCP level as well.

Additional considerations must be taken into account. Coronal plane balance and joint stability must be assessed clinically and radiographically. Naturally, severe contractures with the finger in the palm are challenging to assess on exam and via radiographs, and must be evaluated on a case-by-case basis. Evaluation of overall gross joint alignment may be all that is possible in these scenarios. Joints with collateral ligament insufficiency and coronal plane imbalance should not be treated with continuous extension torque, as the force vectors will not remain balanced along the joint's sagittal plane flexion-extension axis. The phalangeal bone itself must be evaluated. Phalangeal fractures have been reported after manipulation treatment for Dupuytren's contracture; therefore, phalangeal bone quality should be evaluated for osteopenia or osteoporosis as this may increase the risk for fracture and/or pin loosening [18]. Prior deformity or fracture malunion may force an out-of-plane trajectory of the pin correction axis, thereby negating potential benefits of the extension torque. Presence of advanced arthritic joint degeneration or bone loss may render the outcome less effective and may lead to increased pain from a now more mobile arthritic joint. Finally, akin to any elective surgical intervention, the presence of overlying infection or skin compromise should be permitted to resolve prior to treatment.

Further patient factors to consider include history of prior finger and hand trauma or surgery. Pre-existing flexor tendon injury, scarring and adhesions, pulley injuries, or prior surgical scarring can increase the risk of recurrent contracture [19, 20]. These are not contraindications, but rather are important factors to discuss with patients during pre-operative counseling and expectation management. Additionally, the ability and willingness to participate in regular hand therapy is beneficial to a successful outcome, and this must be emphasized to patients pre-operatively [21].

Patient psychology is another essential component to successful treatment. Some patients are simply less tolerant of external fixation and the necessary daily maintenance and hygiene required for this method of treatment [22]. In this vein, patients must fully "buy in" to the treatment and be capable of understanding their part in the gradual progressive correction. Many devices require adjustment of flexible bands of differing strengths, turning and advancement of fixator dials to increase extension torque, removal and correct replacement of hand-based orthoses during daily hygiene, pin site care, etc. Patients that cannot comply with these components of care are at increased risk of poor outcome. Additionally, patients with underlying spasticity present a unique challenge, not only regarding continuous extension torque but for Dupuytren's treatment in general [23]. It is prudent in these patients to fully investigate the etiology of spasticity and attempt some treatment to ameliorate this prior to proceeding with continuous extension torque.

As previously mentioned, specifics of technique and instrumentation vary depending on the device chosen. One of the most popular devices in the United States is the Digit Widget, developed by Dr. John Agee and the Hand Biomechanics Lab in Sacramento, CA. Given the ease and reproducibility of application, simple instrumentation, and straightforward post-operative management during the correction period, its popularity is not surprising. In addition to the technique by Agee and Goss [17], The Hand Biomechanics Lab [24] and the American Academy of Orthopaedic Surgeons Orthopaedic Video Theater (AAOS OVT) [25] offer thorough, step-wise videos of device application with illustrative cases.

In brief, the technique involves placing the patient supine with the hand on an arm board. Digital nerve blockade, with or without supplementary anesthesia, is utilized. The pin targeting guide is placed atop the dorsal aspect of the middle phalanx, and using fluoroscopy Kirschner wires are advanced bi-cortically. These are then removed and replaced by the threaded pins until the far cortex is just engaged. The coupling device is secured to the pins and the hand-based orthotic strap is placed. Flexible bands are then applied between the coupling device and the hand-based orthosis, completing the procedure. The device is to be worn as often as possible daily, with removal of the hand straps recommended solely for daily hand hygiene. Other proprietary devices or make-shift external fixators essentially follow similar surgical steps, with initial bony fixation into the phalanx and some method of attachment to a hand-based accessory for correction.

Length of continuous extension torque treatment varies by patient, depending on the extent of contracture, compliance with necessary torque adjustments, and ability to tolerate long-duration daily wear. Typical duration of treatment is between 6 and 8 weeks, and an average weekly 10–20° extension improvement can occur. However, it is important to discuss variability in time frame with patients pre-operatively. Additional attention to the MCP joint during treatment is crucial to avoid unintended MCP hyperextension. If this is noted during the course, treatment can be adjusted and a supplemental strap can be used for MCP flexion. Patients should be regularly monitored during the treatment duration to ensure appropriate progression of correction, adjustment of torque rubber bands as needed, management of hand edema, skin assessment, and monitoring of any issues such as off-axis strap positioning that can begin turning the fingers if not recognized and addressed.

The end of the treatment period occurs when either the finger has achieved full extension, or once the extension correction plateaus after several weeks. At this stage, one of two paths is taken. The device can be simply removed in the office, followed by regular combination of hand therapy, home exercises, and night-time extension orthosis to maintain the correction. Alternatively, the second stage surgery can then be scheduled and performed, involving device removal and partial palmar fasciectomy (preferred authors algorithm).

9.3 Evidence-Based Outcomes

The literature for evaluation of the effect of continuous extension torque on Dupuytren's contracture correction is overall limited. However, the available studies appear to demonstrate overall promising and potentially beneficial outcomes compared to traditional fasciectomy alone.

In a study comparing initial soft tissue distraction using the Digit Widget followed by open fasciectomy versus open fasciectomy and checkrein ligament release, Craft et al. [15] demonstrated superior outcomes in the preliminary distraction group. The fasciectomy and checkrein release group had initial mean PIP joint flexion contracture of 55.9° corrected by an average of 37.4°. In contrast, the distraction plus fasciectomy group had initial mean PIP joint flexion contracture of 67.6° corrected by an average of 54.8°. Three of the 17 digits in the distraction group corrected completely at the end of the distraction phase, and did not require fasciectomy. At mean follow-up of 18 months, neither group demonstrated recurrence or loss of the gained extension. These results are overall promising for correction of severe PIP joint contractures. But it is important to note that the mean follow-up period of 18 months is relatively short. Additionally, the distraction group demonstrated four complications unique to external fixation usage. One patient required early device removal due to neighboring digit impingement. Another patient experienced MCP hyperextension requiring a blocking splint. Two patients suffered pin tract infections managed with antibiotics. It is prudent to discuss the unique possible complications of external fixation, whether minor or potentially severe, with patients pre-operatively.

The effect of staged treatment with initial external extension fixation followed by open fasciectomy was further studied by Qui et al. [16] They found a mean improvement in PIP joint flexion contracture from 81° to 23° following staged management. At an average follow-up of 15 months, the mean residual PIP joint flexion contracture was 39°. Although this did show some recurrence of PIP joint contracture, the authors found no differences in patient-reported outcome scores based on the amount of flexion contracture recurrence.

Utilizing a different device, the TEC, Messina et al. [26] assessed the corrective potential of the external torque device alone versus initial external extension torque followed by open fasciectomy. Of the 85 total fingers treated, 23 were managed with TEC device alone while 62 fingers were treated with TEC followed by open fasciectomy. They found that the TEC alone group demonstrated rapid progression of flexion contracture by 10 days following removal. However, the group with subsequent open fasciectomy exhibited lower rates of recurrent contracture at 5 years post-operatively. In addition to lower recurrence with staged treatment, they found the fasciectomy itself was easier in terms of skin incisions and approach, faster surgical time, and decreased the need for adjunct procedures such as skin grafts.

In another study, Citron et al. [10] retrospectively reviewed their experience with 18 fingers managed with staged initial external fixation to apply extension torque, followed by open fasciectomy. At 18 months follow-up, they observed a mean correction of PIP joint flexion contracture from 80° pre-operatively to 29°, with three patients experiencing recurrent contracture. Interestingly, they used two different external fixation devices, the TEC and Verona, in their patients. However, they reported inadequate numbers to comment on possible device-related differences. In contrast, Hodgkinson [11] retrospectively reported on external extension torque alone, without fasciectomy, using a device called the PIPSTER. In seven treated fingers of five patients, they found an average 45° improvement of PIP joint flexion contracture. The number of treated patients was of course quite low, and they further did not comment on outcomes of the subsequent surgical fasciectomies that were performed. Beard and Trail [27] utilized continuous extension torque in a different method, applying it after surgical fasciectomy in 18 patients. They ultimately found disappointing results, with only five of 18 treated fingers maintaining improved results.

Ultimately, the literature highlights a dearth of high-level, comparative assessment of the effect of continuous extension torque for Dupuytren's contracture correction. The presented studies illustrate promising results in terms of contracture correction, particularly when combined with subsequent open fasciectomy. Several factors should be considered when interpreting the results and also when considering future directions for investigation. Prospective studies are currently lacking and are needed to properly elucidate the effect of extension torque treatment for severe Dupuytren's cases. Overall patient numbers and length of follow-up are both low. Organizing multi-center trials with long-duration assessment of contracture recurrence and patient-reported outcomes will better inform surgeons of longer-term treatment expectations. These larger studies may be able to further provide granular data regarding possible cut-off values for degrees of contracture, and the expected long-term improvement with versus without initial external fixation. Finally, the majority of current studies focus solely on PIP joint contracture and correction; however, very severe cases also involve MCP joint contracture. Understanding the potential ability or limitations of continuous extension torque in cases of severe combined PIP and MCP flexion contractures will provide further clinical insight for these challenging cases.

References

1. Jones NF, Huang JI. Emergency microsurgical revascularization for critical ischemia during surgery for Dupuytren's contracture: a case report. J Hand Surg Am. 2001;26:1125.
2. Eberlin KR, Mudgal CS. Complications of treatment for Dupuytren disease. Hand Clin. 2018;34:387.
3. Boyer MI, Gelberman RH. Complications of the operative treatment of Dupuytren's disease. Hand Clin. 1999;15:161.
4. Ball C, Izadi D, Verjee LS, Chan J, Nanchahal J. Systematic review of non-surgical treatments for early dupuytren's disease. BMC Musculoskelet Disord. 2016;17:345.
5. Hurst LC, Badalamente MA. Nonoperative treatment of Dupuytren's disease. Hand Clin. 1999;15:97.
6. Rayan GM. Nonoperative treatment of Dupuytren's disease. J Hand Surg Am. 2008;33:1208.
7. Corain M, Zanotti F, Sartore R, Pozza P. Proposal for treatment of severe Dupuytren disease in 2 steps: progressive distraction with external fixator and collagenase – a preliminary case series. Hand. 2020;15:631.
8. Zolotov AS. Two-stage treatment of severe Dupuytren's contracture with an external fixator. J Hand Surg Eur. 2020;45:301.
9. Messina A, Messina J. The TEC treatment (continuous extension technique) for severe Dupuytren's contracture of the fingers. Ann Chir Main Memb Super. 1991;10(3):247–50.
10. Citron N, Messina JC. The use of skeletal traction in the treatment of severe primary Dupuytren's disease. J Bone Joint Surg Br. 1998;80:126.
11. Hodgkinson PD. The use of skeletal traction to correct the flexed PIP joint in Dupuytren's disease. A pilot study to assess the use of the Pipster. J Hand Surg. 1994;19:534.
12. Kasabian A, McCarthy J, Karp N. Use of a multiplanar distracter for the correction of a proximal interphalangeal joint contracture. Ann Plast Surg. 1998;40:378.
13. Kasparyan NG, Hotchkiss RN. Dynamic skeletal fixation in the upper extremity. Hand Clin. 1997;13:643.
14. Rajesh KR, Rex C, Mehdi H, Martin C, Fahmy NRM. Severe Dupuytren's contracture of the proximal interphalangeal joint: treatment by two-stage technique. J Hand Surg. 2000;25:442.
15. Craft RO, Smith AA, Coakley B, Casey WJ III, Rebecca AM, Duncan SF. Preliminary soft-tissue distraction versus checkrein ligament release after fasciectomy in the treatment of dupuytren proximal interphalangeal joint contractures. Plast Reconstr Surg. 2011;128:1107.
16. Qiu B, Hammert W, Wilbur D. External fixation prior to fasciectomy leads to substantial improvement of advanced Dupuytren's PIP contractures at mean follow-up 15 months. Hand. 2023;19:1293.
17. Agee JM, Goss BC. The use of skeletal extension torque in reversing Dupuytren contractures of the proximal interphalangeal joint. J Hand Surg Am. 2012;37:1467.
18. Lewallen LW, Rizzo M. Phalangeal fracture during attempted Dupuytrens release following clostridial collagenase injection: case report. J Orthop Case Rep. 2017;7

19. Radhamony NG, Nair RR, Sreenivasan S, Walkay S, Soni A, Kakkar R. Residual deformity versus recurrence following Dupuytren's palmar fasciectomy-a long term follow-up of 142 cases. Ann Med Surg. 2022;73:103224.
20. Dias JJ, Singh HP, Ullah A, Bhowal B, Thompson JR. Patterns of recontracture after surgical correction of Dupuytren disease. J Hand Surg Am. 2013;38:1987.
21. Skirven TM, Bachoura A, Jacoby SM, Culp RW, Osterman AL. The effect of a therapy protocol for increasing correction of severely contracted proximal interphalangeal joints caused by dupuytren disease and treated with collagenase injection. J Hand Surg Am. 2013;38:684.
22. Abulaiti A, Yilihamu Y, Yasheng T, Alike Y, Yusufu A. The psychological impact of external fixation using the Ilizarov or Orthofix LRS method to treat tibial osteomyelitis with a bone defect. Injury. 2017;48:2842.
23. Beecher SM, Lane O'Neill B, O'Shaughnessy M. Collagenase use and a trap for the unwary in patients with upper limb spasticity. Hand. 2021;16:832.
24. Agee J, Hand Biomechanics Lab, Instructional Video Agee Digit Widget, https://handbiolab.com/digit-widget/, November 2023.
25. Toston RJ, Dawes AM, Gottschalk MB, Hurt JT, Karzon A, Ojemakinde AA, Stewart C, Wagner ER. The Use of the Agee Digit Widget (Continuous Extension Technique) for Extreme Dupuytrens PIP Contractures. AAOS OVT, https://www.aaos.org/videos/video-detail-page/25495__Videos, March 15th, 2022.
26. Messina A, Messina J. The continuous elongation treatment by the TEC device for severe Dupuytren's contracture of the fingers. Plast Reconstr Surg. 1993;92:84.
27. Beard AJ, Trail IA. The "S" Quattro in severe Dupuytren's contracture. J Hand Surg. 1996;21:795.

Chapter 10
Dupuytren Disease: Considerations in Revision Intervention

Sanjeev Kakar and Sarah Townsley

10.1 How to Define Recurrent Dupuytren Disease

Dupuytren disease (DD) is a disorder of cellular hyperproliferation with a tendency to recur after treatment. A wide range of recurrence rates of DD after initial treatment have been reported in the literature, with rates varying between% 0 and 100% [3]. Inconsistent definitions of recurrence have contributed to this variability. A literature review from 2013 found that only 49% of 113 articles discussing recurrence rates of DD provided a definition and that three different types of recurrence were used in the literature [3]. Type I recurrence was defined as return of disease in the form of nodules or cords in the operative area or hand. Type II recurrence was defined as presence of contracture with as little as 1° considered recurrence. Type III recurrence was defined as a patient-reported recurrence.

To help improve discussions on DD recurrence clinically and in research, two separate, independent, international consensus study groups met to develop a consensus definition of DD recurrence. Both study groups used the Delphi method and came to similar conclusions about how to define DD recurrence. Felici et al. [4] stated that a time 0 measurement should be made at 6 weeks to 3 months postoperatively to serve as a baseline whereafter recurrence is defined as a passive extension deficit increase of greater than 20° in at least one treated joint compared to baseline in the presence of a palpable cord. Kan et al. [5] defined recurrence as greater than 20° of contracture in any single treated joint at 1 year post-treatment compared to 6 weeks post-treatment. Both definitions were similar but differed on the time point of follow-up and presence of a palpable cord.

S. Kakar (✉) · S. Townsley
Mayo Clinic, Rochester, MN, USA
e-mail: Kakar.Sanjeev@mayo.edu

M. B. Gottschalk et al. (eds.), *Dupuytren's Disease*,
https://doi.org/10.1007/978-3-031-85873-4_10

10.2 Preoperative Assessment

When a patient presents with recurrent DD, several factors must be considered when determining the best treatment approach. The surgeon must consider the patients' goals and preferences, the prior surgeries that have been performed, and the time to recurrence. This information should be gathered when taking the patient history, along with results and complications from their initial treatment and other areas of disease.

The physical exam provides important insights into the best course of treatment for the patient. The surgeon must assess the nature of the recurrence, for example, whether it is the result of recurrent fibromatosis or if it is the result of secondary contractures involving the joint and its surrounding structures. The hand should be examined for skin quality, neurovascular status, cords and nodules, and surgical incision and passive extension deficit (PED) or range of motion should be measured at all involved joints. Adaptive changes should be appreciated, including joint contractures and boutonniere deformity.

During the course of the history, it is important to elucidate the treatment undertaken for primary disease as this may impact the outcome after treatment for recurrence. Mendelaar et al. [2] performed a retrospective review which found that, compared to patients whose initial treatment was limited fasciectomy, those who underwent initial treatment with needle aponeurotomy had better outcomes in terms of contracture reduction after reoperation with limited fasciectomy. They noted a contracture reduction of 40° in those who underwent initial needle aponeurotomy compared to a contracture reduction of 24° in those who underwent initial limited fasciectomy. Wong et al. [6] performed a review of patients who underwent treatment for recurrent DD. Contrary to the results found by Mendelaar et al. [2], Wong et al. found that the effects of previous treatment on success of revision treatment were unknown. They do note that when prior surgical treatment has been performed, neurovascular structures can be embedded in scar tissue, leading to difficulty with dissection. However, they note that collagenase injections have also been found to alter the microscopic and macroscopic environment of the palm and finger, leading to difficulty with dissection. Despite these theoretical risks, they did not find any studies that supported an increased risk of neurovascular injury after recurrent treatment in this setting. In contrast, a literature review by Denkler et al. [7] assessed complication rates after primary and recurrent DD treatment and found that incidence of neurovascular injury was 10 times higher for recurrent disease than primary disease, occurring in 20% of cases for recurrent disease but only 2% of cases for primary disease, though this was not statistically significant.

Certain factors in the patient's history and physical may indicate an increased risk of recurrence or reoperation. Dupuytren diathesis has been shown to increase the risk of recurrent disease [8]. Dupuytren diathesis is a term that refers to certain features of DD and indicates a more aggressive form of the disease and has been defined as family history with one or more affected siblings or parents, age of onset less than 50 years, male gender, bilateral disease and ectopic disease in the knuckles. It has been found that having presence of all five of these factors increases the risk of recurrence by 71% compared to a baseline risk of 23% in the absence of these factors [8]. Patients should also be aware of a higher rate of recurrence with involvement of the PIP joint due to contracture of the volar plate and collateral ligaments followed by central slip attenuation, making it harder to maintain extension of the PIP joint especially for prolonged contractures [9]. Based on a longitudinal population-based cohort study using a National Health Service (NHS) linked database, Alser et al. [10] identified risk factors for reoperation on the same hand within 10 years of the index surgery. Probability of reoperation was 19.5% after limited fasciectomy, 18.2% after dermofasciectomy, and 33.7% after percutaneous needle aponeurotomy. Risk of reoperation was found to be higher for women and younger patients in some studies, however, other studies have found the opposite results. Hozack et al. [11] performed a retrospective review of all surgeries performed for recurrent DD over a 40—year period. They noted that those who underwent surgery for recurrent disease were more often men (84%) with an average age of 60 years. Many patients undergoing revision surgery had involvement of the small finger (75%) and PIP joint (82%).

10.3 Treatment for Recurrent Disease

When considering revision surgery for DD, it is important to remember that the goal of intervention is to control symptoms of the disease, not cure the disease, and recurrence is high. Treatment for recurrent DD can be challenging, and no single best treatment modality is agreed upon in the literature. Treatment decisions should be individualized to the patient, including their current anatomy, goals and prior treatments. Hozack et al. [12] performed a retrospective review of treatment for recurrent DD. They noted that the most common procedure performed for recurrent DD was partial fasciectomy (72%), followed by dermofasciectomy (23%), radical fasciectomy (6%), needle aponeurotomy (2%), PIP arthrodesis (2%), and ray amputation (2%). They noted that nearly half of their patients undergoing treatment for recurrent disease required full-thickness skin grafting. They also noted that patients with small finger disease with a spiral cord and severe PIP joint contracture may have involvement of their cord with the neurovascular structures leading to incomplete release and higher likelihood for recurrence. Wong et al. [6] performed a systematic review and meta-analysis which demonstrated that the most common treatment for recurrence at 56.6% of all treatments was an open procedure, such as aponeurotomy, dermofasciectomy, or limited fasciectomy, followed by percutaneous needle aponeurotomy at 21.9%, CCH injection at 17%, ray or digit amputation at 2.6%, and PIP arthrodesis at 2.0%. Open fasciectomy sometimes required supplementary procedures to obtain correction, such as interphalangeal arthrodesis (3.4%), PIP joint release (14.8%), and local skin graft or flap (19.3%).

Previous studies have attempted to help guide the surgeon on what to expect after surgery for recurrent disease. Overall, Mendelaar et al. [2] found that treatment for recurrent disease was as effective as treatment for primary disease. A systematic review and meta-analysis by Wong et al. [6] found that overall, treatment of recurrent disease led to a ROM improvement of 23.3° for the MCP joint and 15° for the PIP joint. Given that the minimum clinically important difference (MCID) was found to be 13.5°, this represented a clinically significant improvement. Additional recurrence after this treatment was noted in 20.7% of patients. When looking specifically at the PIP joint, they found that overall, the pooled results demonstrated achievement of MCID improvement in range of motion after all treatment modalities without one procedure deemed more effective than another. Despite these good results, PIP joint contractures can be challenging to maintain correction. During open surgery, release of the volar plate and collateral ligaments helps with immediate improvement of the contracture but can lead to stiffness secondary to swelling and scar formation within the digit. Additionally, long-standing central slip attenuation may lead to difficulty with extension of the joint [9]. Overall, the most common treatment for recurrent disease is partial fasciectomy, and good results can be seen following treatment for recurrent disease though it may be more challenging with higher risk of neurovascular injury.

10.4 Percutaneous Needle Aponeurotomy

Percutaneous techniques, including needle aponeurotomy, can be considered as a revision technique in a patient with a palpable cord or well-defined recurrent disease. This technique is indicated when there is greater MCP than PIP involvement and is contraindicated when scar tissues prevent palpation of the cord and if there is prior neurovascular compromise that impairs the surgeon's ability to assess neurovascular status during the procedure [13]. In the presence of severe contractures, a percutaneous technique will not be able to address secondary structures contributing to the contracture. Van Rijssen and Werker published a retrospective review of a 30 patients series in which 40 fingers with recurrent Dupuytren disease were treated with percutaneous needle aponeurotomy after prior treatment with either percutaneous needle aponeurotomy or limited fasciotomy [1]. They found that there was no difference in contracture reduction when percutaneous needle aponeurotomy was performed as the revision surgery regardless of whether the primary surgery was needle aponeurotomy or limited fasciotomy. They found a reduction in the passive extension deficit in the metacarpophalangeal (MCP) joint of 93% and 57% in the proximal interphalangeal (PIP) joint, which was statistically significant. At an average follow-up of 4.4 years, 50% of patients developed re-contracture which was treated with limited fasciotomy at an average of 1.4 years after their first revision procedure. They concluded, based on these results, that percutaneous needle fasciotomy delayed the need for limited fasciotomy by 2.9 years on average. There were no serious adverse events. They stated that percutaneous needle fasciotomy allows for a fast recovery with minimal complications, but may lead to relatively early recurrence in half of patients. In our experience, the use of continuous skeletal

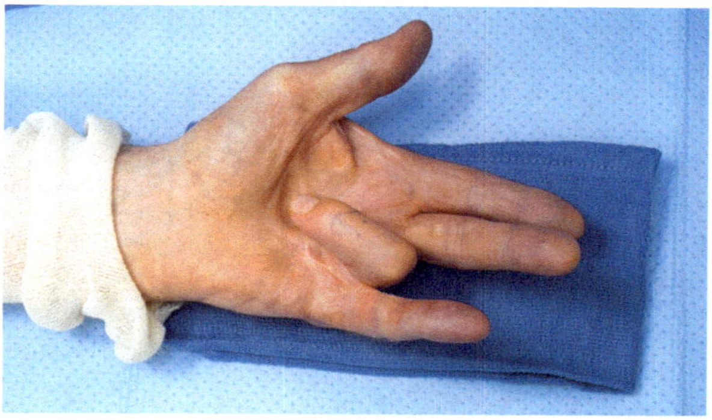

Fig. 10.1 Demonstrates flexion contracture of the ring finger with recurrent Dupuytren disease

extension torque devices or temporary K wire fixation of the PIPJ in a more extended position can be used in conjunction with needle aponeurotomy in the setting of a PIP joint contracture. After performing the needle aponeurotomy, there can be scarring or contracture of the volar plate of the PIP joint leading to continued contracture. The use of the continuous skeletal extension torque device can then be used to provide slow elongation of this structure and improve the PIP joint contracture. Another way in which the continuous passive elongation device is used in conjunction with needle aponeurotomy is in a staged fashion before an open procedure. A surgeon can perform needle aponeurotomy and place a device in the same episode to provide some immediate correction, then proceed with an open procedure 4–8 weeks later with removal of the device [9].

We present an illustrative case example of how PIP joint pinning in conjunction with needle aponeurotomy can be used in the revision setting. Our first case is a patient who developed recurrent contracture in his ring finger 14 years after undergoing palmar fasciectomy and presented 4 years after his recurrence. On his presentation with recurrence, his MCP range of motion was from 70° to 75° and his PIP range of motion was from 90° to 95° (Fig. 10.1). He underwent needle aponeurotomy with temporary extension pinning of his PIP joint. At his 3-month follow-up, his MCP range of motion improved to 5–90° and his PIP range of motion improved to 20–90° (Fig. 10.2a, b).

10.5 Clostridium Histolyticum Injection

Clostridium histolyticum (CCH) injection is an option for patients with recurrent disease regardless of their initial treatment for DD except for those who previously demonstrated a hypersensitivity reaction to the injection [13]. Additionally, caution should be used when considering this technique in patients with prior local skin graft, as skin graft loss has previously been demonstrated [14]. This technique is preferred in the setting of limited scarring and with a clearly defined cord. Bear et al. previously investigated the effectiveness of CCH in patients with recurrent DD

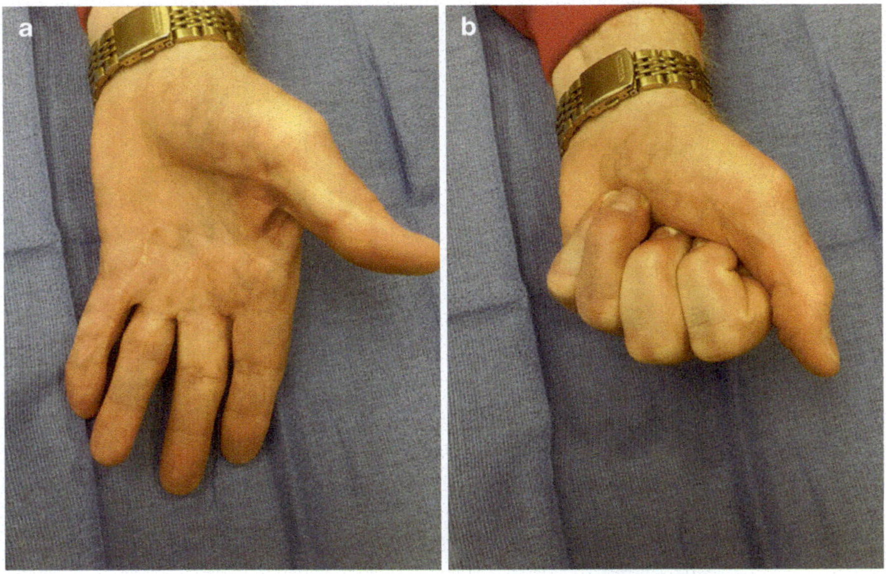

Fig. 10.2 (**a** and **b**): Demonstrates appearance of the ring finger at the 3-month postoperative visit in extension (**a**) and flexion (**b**)

who were previously treated with CCH [15]. They performed an open-label phase 4 study of patients who previously participated in the Collagenase Option for Reduction of Dupuytren Long-Term Evaluation of Safety Study (CORDLESS) and were previously effectively treated with CCH and developed a palpable cord with increase in contracture of 20° or more compared with 30 days post treatment. 57% of the patients in their study achieved a fixed flexion contracture at the treated joint of 5° or less. The percentage of patients who achieved this degree of contracture improvement was higher in MCP joints at 65% compared to PIP joints at 45%. There was no increase in adverse effects compared to initial treatment. Bainbridge et al. assessed the efficacy of CCH for recurrent contracture in the setting of prior surgical intervention for DD [16]. They analyzed a group of 1082 patients who received CCH injection, 40% of whom had received prior surgery for DD and compared them to the patients in that group who had not received prior surgery. The previously operated group underwent treatment with CCH an average of 5 years after surgical treatment. There was no significant difference in range of motion or fixed flexion contracture of the MCP or PIP joint after CCH in patients previously treated with surgery compared to those never treated with surgery. They found that previously operated hands had a higher rate of adverse events as well as serious adverse events. Serious adverse events in the previously operated hands include tendon ruptures, deep vein thrombosis of the lower extremity, and tendonitis. Non-serious adverse events that were more common in the previously operated hand included peripheral edema, contusions, ecchymosis, pain, tenderness, and lymphadenopathy.

10.6 Limited Fasciectomy

Open fasciectomy maybe considered in all cases of recurrent DD and is considered the gold standard [13]. It is particularly indicated in the setting of significant scarring, a poorly palpable cord, and distorted anatomy. Great care is needed when performing this procedure as PIP joint contractures of 60° have been found to increase the risk of surgical complications, and could be considered an indicator of severe disease [17].

Several studies have evaluated the outcomes of open fasciectomy for recurrent DD. Konneker et al. evaluated 16 patients with history of severe DD who had undergone at least 2 prior surgeries on the same hand for DD and presented to their clinic where they underwent a third surgical intervention for DD [18]. They found a patient satisfaction rate of 76.9% despite 64.3% of patients with extension deficits remaining after treatment. They demonstrated a mean improvement for the PIP joint of 59.2° and 86.2%. No recurrences were found after 40 months of follow-up using the definition put forth by Felici et al. One severe complication was observed, which was finger amputation due to osteomyelitis due to delayed K-wire extraction. They report that the benefit of open fasciectomy compared to percutaneous techniques is the ability to address and repair neurovascular injuries if they occur. They suggest that based on the results of their study, repeated limited fasciectomy is an acceptable treatment option for patients who have had prior surgeries.

Spies et al. performed a retrospective analysis of 18 patients with recurrent DD who underwent treatment with open partial aponeurectomy [19]. 36% of fingers experienced a recurrent contracture with recurrence defined based on the definition by van Rijssen et al. [20] 83% of patients had a grip strength of 90% or higher compared to their contralateral side. 56% of patients had a pinch strength of 90% or higher compared to their contralateral side. 83% of patients had a disabilities of arm, shoulder, and hand (DASH) score 15 or lower, which is considered excellent. 56% of patients had no pain. 56% of patients had an improved outcome whereas 44% were not satisfied. Severe complications did not occur, however there was a fifth ray amputation due to PIP joint subluxation/fracture that was thought to be unrelated to the procedure. They concluded that open limited aponeurectomy is a safe and effective procedure for recurrent DD.

Eberlin et al. specifically evaluated the outcome of digital or palmar fasciectomy after prior treatment with CCH [21]. The average time from CCH injection to salvage fasciectomy was 12 months. Intraoperatively, it was noted that normal tissue architecture was disrupted, and extensive scar tissue was present in the dissection planes. Histologically, these changes are indistinguishable from tissue seen in prior fasciectomy [22]. In a survey of clinicians who performed surgical fasciectomy after CCH injection, 7 out of 9 surgeons felt that there was no significant distortion of anatomy and felt that the technical difficulty was equivalent to a primary Dupuytren surgery whereas one surgeon reported significant increased difficulty and distorted anatomy [23]. Despite possible increased technical difficulty, significant improvement in range of motion was seen postoperatively and the authors note that the results are comparable to those seen after primary fasciectomy.

Early studies of open fasciectomy noted that surgery for recurrent disease was associated with a higher rate of neurovascular injury, with a 3.9% risk in primary procedures and a 57.7% risk in surgery for recurrent disease [24]. In this same study, there also appeared to be a higher rate of stiffness in patients who underwent surgery for recurrent disease [24]. A more recent literature review comparing complications of primary and recurrent diseases found that overall, complication rates for primary disease (30.8%) are higher than those with recurrent disease (25%) [7]. However, they noted a ten-fold higher rate of digital nerve and artery injuries in patients with recurrent disease (approximately 20%) compared to primary disease (approximately 2%) [7].

10.7 Dermofasciectomy

Dermofasciectomy can be considered for recurrent disease in the presence of widespread scarring and fibrosis where a cord is not easily palpable. Additionally, this technique can be considered in the setting of significant PIP joint contracture [13]. Dermofasciectomy has been described for both primary and recurrent disease. Dermofasciectomy was described by Hueston et al. for the treatment of both primary and recurrent DD in 1969 [25]. He described the use in primary disease for those in which he deemed recurrence highly likely, such as a young patient with rapidly progressive disease or significant Dupuytren diathesis. He noted no recurrences in his study cohort. Additionally, Brotherston et al. [26] reported their results of 34 patients who underwent dermofasciectomy and full-thickness skin graft for recurrent disease in a 1994 review. Their patient cohort had an average follow-up of 80–120 months. They reported no evidence of recurrence in the region of their skin grafts at follow-up.

Subsequent studies have not found such promising results after dermofasciectomy for recurrent DD. Roush and Stern reported on their results of dermofasciectomy for recurrent DD when compared to limited fasciectomy and interphalangeal (IP) arthrodesis and fasciectomy with a local flap [27]. They found that patients who underwent dermofasciectomy did not have statistically significant improvements in total active motion at follow-up compared to preoperative motion, whereas patients who underwent fasciectomy and a local flap did experience statistically significant improvements in total active motion.

10.8 Joint Arthrodesis

Joint arthrodesis can be considered for severe, recurrent PIP joint contracture in the setting of DD. This is typically only considered after at least two revision procedures and as an alternative to revision fasciectomy, dermofasciectomy, or digit amputation. There are various techniques that have been described to achieve fusion of the digit and improvement of the contracture. Bolt et al. [28] reported on a series of 11 patients who underwent PIP joint fusion with concomitant needle or open fasciectomy as treatment for their third recurrence of DD. A majority of patients underwent the procedure in their small finger but one patient did undergo the procedure in their ring finger. They performed the fasciectomy in order to achieve straightening of the digit without having to excise additional bone. There was a mean follow-up of 8 years and 9 months. They found that arthrodesis was achieved in all patients. All patients reported that they were able to carry out all of their activities of daily living and return to work if applicable. Patients reported that their recovery and return to activities after the arthrodesis was faster than their prior surgeries. No complications were reported. In a series of 11 patients by Watson and Lovallo in 1987 [29], they performed PIP arthrodesis without fasciectomy and instead performed shortening of the proximal phalanx for deformity correction in the small and ring finger. Using this technique, they achieved an angle of 30° in the small finger and 37° in the ring finger. Two of their patients noted that the shortened digit made it harder to hold objects in the ulnar side of the palm.

Resection of the middle phalanx to achieve deformity correction has also been described by multiple authors as an alternative to amputation for recurrent disease of the small finger. The shortening arthrodesis was originally described by Honecker et al. in 2016 [30] in a 7-patient series in which the middle phalanx was removed through a dorsal approach and the proximal and distal phalanx were fused. They found that all digits fused and there was improvement in pain and QuickDASH scores. One patient experienced cold intolerance. Vanmierlo et al. published a modification of the Honecker technique in 2023 [31] in which a volar aponeurectomy was performed in addition to the middle phalanx excision. In their 13-patient series, at a mean follow-up of 124 days, 11 patients were able to achieve full MP joint extension and full small finger adduction. Mean MP joint flexion was 93°, and there was improvement in QuickDASH scores from 19.6 preoperatively to 11.6 postoperatively. Pain scores remained unchanged between pre and postoperative measurements.

Another alternative to amputation for small finger PIP joint contractures described by Eiriksdottir et al. [32] involves resection of the middle phalanx and ligament reconstruction to create a new interphalangeal joint between the proximal and distal phalanx. Results from their procedure performed for two patients demonstrated near full extension, normal sensation, and no pain with active flexion to 60 and 35° at the IP joint and full MCP range of motion.

10.9 Ray/Digit Amputation

Digit amputation can be considered for refractory Dupuytren contracture that is severely interfering with hand function. Degreef et al. [33] noted that elective amputation for DD accounts for 39% of all elective amputations and all of these occurred in the fourth or fifth ray. In their series, they also found that elective amputation accounts for 2% of all surgical procedures performed for DD. They found that function was similar to that seen after post-traumatic amputation.

Jensen et al. [34] reviewed their series of 23 finger amputations in 17 small fingers and six ring fingers. When amputations were performed distal to the MP joint, they found recurrence of lack of extension in 9 out of 16 fingers. When amputations were performed through or proximal to the MP joint, they noted that five out of seven small fingers experienced neuroma or phantom pain.

10.10 Adjunct Procedures

Complication rates with DD surgery have been found to increase with increasing severity of the disease, particularly in patients with PIP joint contractures greater than 60° [17]. With such significant contracture, there can be an increased risk of damage to neurovascular structures during the process of contracture correction or dissection. The use of a Digit Widget can be used to help provide correction of the PIP joint either before or after surgical intervention for DD. It can be staged or can be used in conjunction with a procedure to release the fascia, as its use alone tends to result in recurrence of the contracture. It has been described previously for use in recurrent DD. It has been noted that this typically has good success at improving PIP contracture, but that in the setting of recurrent disease, prior release of the pulleys or joint capsules lead to increased lever arm of the flexor digitorum profundus (FDP) and superficialis (FDS) leading to recurrent contracture [35]. In addition to the above uses, we have used the Digit Widget after needle aponeurotomy for PIP joint contracture to slowly stretch the contracted volar plate and collateral ligaments. It can be used in combination with needle aponeurotomy and an open procedure in a staged fashion. Needle aponeurotomy and the continuous passive elongation device can be applied at a first stage surgery to obtain some correction of the deformity, followed by open fasciectomy 4–8 weeks later with removal of the device [9]. Pinning of the PIP joints can also be used intraoperatively to help maintain improved position of the digit.

Checkrein ligament release can be performed in conjunction with fasciectomy for recurrent disease. In a series by Craft et al. [36] in which checkrein ligament release was performed with fasciectomy for recurrent disease, they found that this procedure worsened two contractures by 3 and 4°, and improved four contractures by a mean of 44°.

Radiation therapy (RT) has a role in treating early-stage DD to prevent disease progression but there have been no studies to date that specifically evaluate radiation therapy for recurrent DD. However, given its use to prevent disease progression [37, 38], it has been considered an option for patients with recalcitrant disease to prevent recurrence, though there is no data to support this in recurrent disease [9].

10.11 Economic Impact

The economic impact of DD is significant given its prevalence and tendency to recur. The estimated treatment cost in England is $52,047,092 over 1 year. Yoon et al. [39] conducted a microsimulation economic analysis to identify cost-effective treatment regimens for recurrent DD. They created a model in which patients underwent a total of 3 surgeries for primary and recurrent DD and calculated the cost based on efficacy of that treatment and severity and location of contracture. They found that for single digits with severe MCP joint contractures, initial treatment with percutaneous needle aponeurotomy followed by limited fasciectomy for recurrence was cost-effective, but that in other joint types, including PIP joint contractures, percutaneous needle aponeurotomy was the only cost-effective treatment for recurrent contractures. However, they do note for that patients whose quality of life is severely affected, limited fasciectomy may be cost-effective for this purpose. CCH was not found to be cost-effective.

10.12 Case Example

We present an illustrative case example of treatment for recurrent DD. The patient had previously undergone needle aponeurotomy for a contracture of his right ring and small finger with recurrence. The ring finger contractures were MCP 45–90, PIP 70–90, DIP 0–30° and small finger was MCP 60–90, PIP 60–90, DIP 0–40° (Fig. 10.3). Given his recurrence with palpable cords, he elected to undergo right ring and small finger palmar fasciectomy and temporary pinning of PIP joint followed by pin removal 4 weeks later. Intraoperatively, the small finger contained a combination of spiral, central, pretendinous, adductor digiti minimi, and lateral digital sheath cords (Fig. 10.4). After identification and protection of the neurovascular bundles with vessel loops, the cords were removed from proximal to distal (Fig. 10.5). After fasciectomy, a PIP joint contracture persisted and thus a volar plate and checkrein ligament release was performed. A similar procedure was performed for the ring finger. Despite correction of the PIPJ contracture, they had a tendency to want to recoil into flexion given their previous long-term contracted state. Therefore, 0.045 K wires were passed temporarily across the PIP joint of the ring and small finger to maintain PIP joint extension and removed several weeks later.

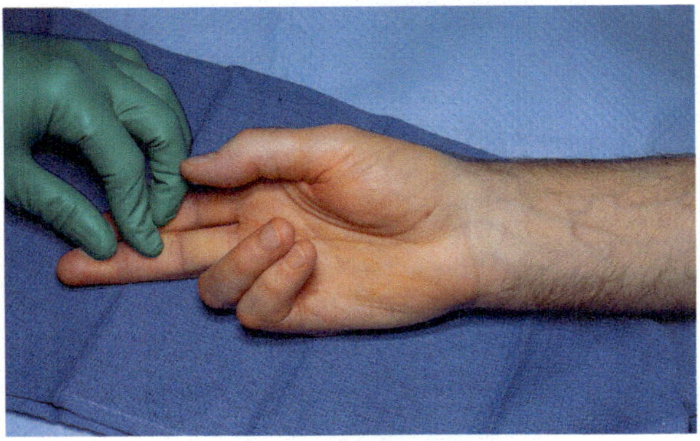

Fig. 10.3 Demonstrates right ring and small finger re-contracture after prior surgical intervention

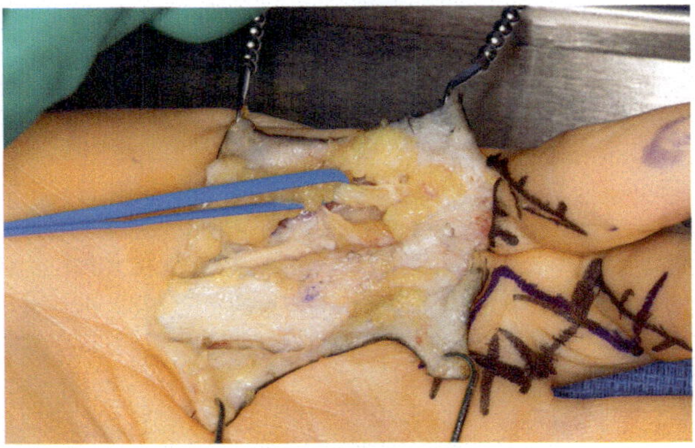

Fig. 10.4 Intraoperative photo demonstrating ulnar neurovascular bundle in blue vessel loop and the cords involving the small finger

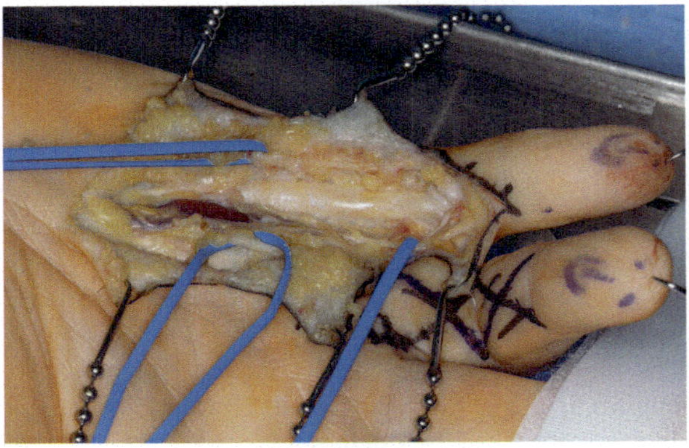

Fig. 10.5 After removal of the cords, one can appreciate the underlying pulleys and flexor tendons with extension of the digit

10.13 Conclusion

Surgical treatment for recurrent DD is safe and effective. The specific treatment modality should be individualized based on the patient's current anatomy, neurovascular status, goals, and preferences for post-treatment recovery. Percutaneous and enzymatic techniques can be used after prior nonsurgical or surgical treatments and are best used in the setting of well-defined, palpable cords. Open techniques, especially limited fasciectomy, can be considered for most cases of recurrence, and are indicated in the setting of diffuse disease, severe contracture or concern for neurovascular status. Continuous passive elongation can be used to help reduce the risk of neurovascular complications and improve contracture. Salvage techniques, including arthrodesis and amputation, can be considered in refractory contractures that severely limit hand function. Percutaneous needle aponeurotomy and limited fasciectomy may be the most cost-effective techniques for recurrent disease.

References

1. van Rijssen AL, Werker PM. Percutaneous needle fasciotomy for recurrent Dupuytren disease. J Hand Surg Am. 2012;37(9):1820–3. https://doi.org/10.1016/j.jhsa.2012.05.022.
2. Mendelaar NHA, Poelstra R, van Nieuwenhoven CA, Slijper HP, Feitz R, Hovius SER, et al. Outcome of recurrent surgery in Dupuytren's disease: comparison with initial treatment. Plast Reconstr Surg. 2019;144(5):828e–35e. https://doi.org/10.1097/prs.0000000000006150.
3. Kan HJ, Verrijp FW, Huisstede BM, Hovius SE, van Nieuwenhoven CA, Selles RW. The consequences of different definitions for recurrence of Dupuytren's disease. J Plast Reconstr Aesthet Surg. 2013;66(1):95–103. https://doi.org/10.1016/j.bjps.2012.08.019.
4. Felici N, Marcoccio I, Giunta R, Haerle M, Leclercq C, Pajardi G, et al. Dupuytren contracture recurrence project: reaching consensus on a definition of recurrence. Handchir Mikrochir Plast Chir. 2014;46(6):350–4. https://doi.org/10.1055/s-0034-1394420.
5. Kan HJ, Verrijp FW, Hovius SER, van Nieuwenhoven CA, Selles RW. Recurrence of Dupuytren's contracture: a consensus-based definition. PLoS One. 2017;12(5):e0164849. https://doi.org/10.1371/journal.pone.0164849.
6. Wong CR, Huynh MNQ, Fageeh R, McRae MC. Outcomes of management of recurrent Dupuytren contracture: a systematic review and meta-analysis. Hand. 2022;17(6):1104–13. https://doi.org/10.1177/1558944721994220.
7. Denkler K. Surgical complications associated with fasciectomy for dupuytren's disease: a 20-year review of the English literature. Eplasty. 2010;10:e15.
8. Hindocha S, Stanley JK, Watson S, Bayat A. Dupuytren's diathesis revisited: evaluation of prognostic indicators for risk of disease recurrence. J Hand Surg Am. 2006;31(10):1626–34. https://doi.org/10.1016/j.jhsa.2006.09.006.
9. Putnam J. Advanced Dupuytren contracture: approach to management. Hand Clin. 2023;39(3):455–63. https://doi.org/10.1016/j.hcl.2023.03.006.
10. Alser O, Craig RS, Lane JCE, Prats-Uribe A, Robinson DE, Rees JL, et al. Serious complications and risk of re-operation after Dupuytren's disease surgery: a population-based cohort study of 121,488 patients in England. Sci Rep. 2020;10(1):16520. https://doi.org/10.1038/s41598-020-73595-y.
11. Hozack BA, Tosti RJ. Fragment-specific fixation in distal radius fractures. Curr Rev Musculoskelet Med. 2019;12(2):190–7. https://doi.org/10.1007/s12178-019-09538-6.

12. Hozack BA, Rayan GM. Surgical treatment for recurrent Dupuytren disease. Hand. 2023;18(4):641–7. https://doi.org/10.1177/15589447211060447.
13. Kaplan FTD, Crosby NE. Treatment of recurrent Dupuytren disease. Hand Clin. 2018;34(3):403–15. https://doi.org/10.1016/j.hcl.2018.03.009.
14. Swanson JW, Watt AJ, Vedder NB. Skin graft loss resulting from collagenase clostridium histolyticum treatment of Dupuytren contracture: case report and review of the literature. J Hand Surg Am. 2013;38(3):548–51. https://doi.org/10.1016/j.jhsa.2012.12.007.
15. Bear BJ, Peimer CA, Kaplan FTD, Kaufman GJ, Tursi JP, Smith T. Treatment of recurrent Dupuytren contracture in joints previously effectively treated with collagenase clostridium histolyticum. J Hand Surg Am. 2017;42(5):391. https://doi.org/10.1016/j.jhsa.2017.02.010.
16. Bainbridge C, Gerber RA, Szczypa PP, Smith T, Kushner H, Cohen B, et al. Efficacy of collagenase in patients who did and did not have previous hand surgery for Dupuytren's contracture. J Plast Surg Hand Surg. 2012;46(3–4):177–83. https://doi.org/10.3109/2000656x.2012.683795.
17. Bulstrode NW, Jemec B, Smith PJ. The complications of Dupuytren's contracture surgery. J Hand Surg Am. 2005;30(5):1021–5. https://doi.org/10.1016/j.jhsa.2005.05.008.
18. Könneker S, Broelsch GF, Krezdorn N, Dastagir K, Kuhbier JW, Paprottka FJ, et al. Multiple recurrences in aggressive forms of Dupuytren's disease-can patients benefit from repeated selective fasciectomy? Plast Reconstr Surg Glob Open. 2017;5(2):e1247. https://doi.org/10.1097/gox.0000000000001247.
19. Spies CK, Hahn P, Müller LP, Löw S, Sellei RM, Oppermann J. The efficacy of open partial aponeurectomy for recurrent Dupuytren's contracture. Arch Orthop Trauma Surg. 2016;136(6):881–9. https://doi.org/10.1007/s00402-016-2448-2.
20. van Rijssen AL, Werker PM. Percutaneous needle fasciotomy in dupuytren's disease. J Hand Surg Br. 2006;31(5):498–501. https://doi.org/10.1016/j.jhsb.2006.03.174.
21. Eberlin KR, Kobraei EM, Nyame TT, Bloom JM, Upton J 3rd. Salvage palmar fasciectomy after initial treatment with collagenase clostridium histolyticum. Plast Reconstr Surg. 2015;135(6):1000e–6e. https://doi.org/10.1097/prs.0000000000001282.
22. Sanjuan-Cervero R, Carrera-Hueso FJ, Vaquero-Perez M, Montaner-Alonso D. Recurrent Dupuytren's disease after fasciectomy and collagenase injection are histologically indistinguishable. J Hand Surg. 2020;45(5):508–12. https://doi.org/10.1177/1753193419900483.
23. Hay DC, Louie DL, Earp BE, Kaplan FT, Akelman E, Blazar PE. Surgical findings in the treatment of Dupuytren's disease after initial treatment with clostridial collagenase (Xiaflex). J Hand Surg Eur. 2014;39(5):463–5. https://doi.org/10.1177/1753193413488305.
24. Sennwald GR. Fasciectomy for treatment of Dupuytren's disease and early complications. J Hand Surg Am. 1990;15(5):755–61. https://doi.org/10.1016/0363-5023(90)90151-G.
25. Hueston JT. The control of recurrent Dupuytren's contracture by skin replacement. Br J Plast Surg. 1969;22(2):152–6. https://doi.org/10.1016/S0007-1226(69)80057-3.
26. Brotherston TM, Balakrishnan C, Milner RH, Brown HG. Long term follow-up of dermofasciectomy for Dupuytren's contracture. Br J Plast Surg. 1994;47(6):440–3. https://doi.org/10.1016/0007-1226(94)90075-2.
27. Roush TF, Stern PJ. Results following surgery for recurrent Dupuytren's disease. J Hand Surg Am. 2000;25(2):291–6. https://doi.org/10.1053/jhsu.2000.jhsu25a0291.
28. Bolt AM, Giele H, McNab ISH, Spiteri M. Outcome of arthrodesis for severe recurrent proximal interphalangeal joint contractures in Dupuytren's disease. J Hand Surg Eur. 2021;46(4):403–5. https://doi.org/10.1177/1753193420960309.
29. Watson HK, Lovallo JL. Salvage of severe recurrent Dupuytren's contracture of the ring and small fingers. J Hand Surg Am. 1987;12(2):287–9. https://doi.org/10.1016/s0363-5023(87)80291-5.
30. Honecker S, Hidalgo Diaz JJ, Naito K, Pire E, Prunières G, Facca S, et al. Proximodistal interphalangeal arthrodesis of the little finger: a series of 7 cases. Hand Surg Rehabil. 2016;35(4):262–5. https://doi.org/10.1016/j.hansur.2016.06.003.
31. Vanmierlo B, Van Eecke E, Decramer A, Vanmierlo T, Van Royen K, Goubau J. Shortening arthrodesis combined with limited fasciectomy in severe recurrent Dupuytren's dis-

ease of the fifth finger. Hand Surg Rehabil. 2023;42(4):291–7. https://doi.org/10.1016/j.hansur.2023.04.005.
32. Eiriksdottir A, Atroshi I. A new finger-preserving procedure as an alternative to amputation in recurrent severe Dupuytren contracture of the small finger. BMC Musculoskelet Disord. 2019;20(1):323. https://doi.org/10.1186/s12891-019-2701-2.
33. Degreef I, De Smet L. Dupuytren's disease: a predominant reason for elective finger amputation in adults. Acta Chir Belg. 2009;109(4):494–7. https://doi.org/10.1080/00015458.2009.11680467.
34. Jensen CM, Haugegaard M, Rasmussen SW. Amputations in the treatment of Dupuytren's disease. J Hand Surg Br. 1993;18(6):781–2. https://doi.org/10.1016/0266-7681(93)90245-b.
35. Agee JM, Goss BC. The use of skeletal extension torque in reversing Dupuytren contractures of the proximal interphalangeal joint. J Hand Surg Am. 2012;37(7):1467–74. https://doi.org/10.1016/j.jhsa.2012.04.023.
36. Craft RO, Smith AA, Coakley B, Casey WJ 3rd, Rebecca AM, Duncan SFM. Preliminary soft-tissue distraction versus checkrein ligament release after fasciectomy in the treatment of dupuytren proximal interphalangeal joint contractures. Plast Reconstr Surg. 2011;128(5):1107–13. https://doi.org/10.1097/PRS.0b013e31822b67c9.
37. Betz N, Ott OJ, Adamietz B, Sauer R, Fietkau R, Keilholz L. Radiotherapy in early-stage Dupuytren's contracture. Long-term results after 13 years. Strahlenther Onkol. 2010;186(2):82–90. https://doi.org/10.1007/s00066-010-2063-z.
38. Kadhum M, Smock E, Khan A, Fleming A. Radiotherapy in Dupuytren's disease: a systematic review of the evidence. J Hand Surg Eur. 2017;42(7):689–92. https://doi.org/10.1177/1753193417695996.
39. Yoon AP, Kane RL, Hutton DW, Chung KC. Cost-effectiveness of recurrent Dupuytren contracture treatment. JAMA Netw Open. 2020;3(10):e2019861. https://doi.org/10.1001/jamanetworkopen.2020.19861.

Chapter 11
When to Amputate

Maureen O'Shaughnessy and Margaux Danby

11.1 Introduction

When addressing Dupuytren's contracture, the primary goal of treatment should be to improve hand function and reduce contracture without resorting to amputation. However, amputation may be a beneficial option for some patients, including those with severe functional impairments, significant contractures not amenable to surgery, significant skin compromise due to ulcers or skin necrosis, recurrences after multiple surgical attempts, and complications from prior procedures. Complications from Dupuytren's disease (DD) and treatment can be very broad and may include persistent contracture and deformity, infection, neurovascular compromise or intractable pain after multiple failed approaches; all of these complications may lead patients to desire amputation. Amputation is often a last resort when a patient's quality of life is significantly compromised, and the decision to proceed with amputation should be shared between the physician and patient after a thorough discussion.

11.2 The Patient Perspective

As Dupuytren's disease progresses, contracture becomes increasingly disabling and interferes with activities of daily living. Function in the affected hand is decreased, limiting a patient's ability to grasp objects and perform fine motor tasks. Moreover, contracture increases the bulk of the hand and limits versatility in shape, making

M. O'Shaughnessy (✉) · M. Danby
University of Kentucky College of Medicine, Lexington, KY, USA
e-mail: meda241@uky.edu

M. B. Gottschalk et al. (eds.), *Dupuytren's Disease*,
https://doi.org/10.1007/978-3-031-85873-4_11

simple actions such as putting the hand in a pocket overly difficult. The flexed finger may also catch on clothing, other body parts such as the eye [1], or other elements in the environment. Perhaps most importantly, flexed digits may be a source of chronic pain for patients. All of these factors may contribute to a patient's decision to seek treatment and consider amputation.

11.3 Considerations for Amputation

Deciding when to amputate digits affected by Dupuytren's disease can be difficult for surgeons and patients. It is important to consider the patient's functionality, desires, medical conditions, and goals. All surgical treatments for Dupuytren's disease carry potential risks of local and systemic complications in addition to the risk of recurrence requiring reoperation following primary surgery. In the literature, primary surgery complication rates for DD are highly variable, with amputation risk as high as 9% in fifth-finger surgery [2]. Given the possibility of eventual amputation for therapeutic benefit, it is important to discuss amputation with patients before initial treatment to ensure they understand amputation is a risk or potential long-term outcome associated with any surgical treatment for Dupuytren's disease [2, 3].

Dupuytren's disease is the most common reason for elective amputation of digits [2]. Amputation is primarily considered in patients with severe disease and contracture. Severe cases may be defined as those with recurrent disease or disabling scar tissue after multiple surgeries; longstanding and progressive disease; neurovascular compromise; high contracture measurement by degrees; the involvement of multiple cords in one digit, multiple joints in one digit, or multiple digits; involvement of the proximal interphalangeal (PIP) joint; and compromised soft tissue coverage.

11.3.1 Primary Treatment Failure

Primary treatments may fail due to the recurrence of the disease itself or due to persistent debility from scar tissue. Greater than 90% of elective amputations for Dupuytren's disease occur in patients with recurrent disease [2]. Recurrence requiring secondary treatment is common, with the 10-year risk of reoperation on the same hand reported at 20% following limited fasciectomy or dermofasciectomy and 33% following percutaneous needle aponeurotomy [4]. Furthermore, the amputation rate for reoperation by limited fasciectomy following dermofasciectomy is especially high (8%), which may reflect the increased risk of surgical disruption of the digital arteries when dissecting through a scarred surgical bed [4].

11.3.2 Dupuytren's Diathesis

Indicators of strong disease diathesis are associated with increased rates of recurrent contracture [1]. These include strong family history, younger age of disease onset, earlier age at first operation, and ectopic deposits. Even if the disease itself does not recur (i.e., contracture of tissue other than the fascia), substantial scar tissue may cause persistent functional difficulty. When poor palmar skin and dense infiltration have exhausted the possibility of palmar surgery, amputation may be the most reasonable treatment option [1].

11.3.3 Longstanding Disease

Longstanding disease over many years may cause severe anatomical injury and change. Neurovascular compromise, as discussed below, may occur due to prolonged contracture of digital nerves and vessels. Longstanding joint contracture can progress to central slip attenuation and resultant boutonniere deformity which is extremely challenging to correct. Contracture can result in autofusion after prolonged involvement, especially at the PIP joint; PIP autofusion and end-stage boutonniere position may lead to amputation being the preferred treatment option [5].

11.3.4 Neurovascular Compromise

Neurovascular compromise is a concern in both recurrent and longstanding disease. In one study, digital nerve injuries and digital artery injuries were approximately ten times more common in patients with recurrent disease (20%) than in those with primary disease (2%), though the size of the study prevented statistical significance [6]. Neurovascular injury due to disease or its treatment may lead to numbness and cold intolerance [3]. Neurovascular damage may also contribute to poor wound healing and surgical complications.

Arterial damage is of particular concern in patients with PIP joint involvement. In an anatomical study of PIP joints in digits amputated due to Dupuytren's disease, all joints studied extended fully after release of accessory collateral ligaments and the volar plate [7]. The first five stages of serial release made no improvement; release of the accessory collateral ligaments was sufficient for most fingers, but two required the release of the origin at the volar plate. The requirement of such an extensive release makes it difficult to preserve the ladder vessels that pass under the checkrein ligaments to supply the flexor tendon via the vinculum [7]. In addition, the lateral and dorsal structures of the digits studied showed severe secondary damage, which may help explain the poor results of corrective surgery in patients with disease involving this joint [7]. Attempts to correct severe flexion contracture of the

PIP joint in patients with recurrent DD can lead to neurovascular compromise requiring elective amputation [5].

11.3.5 Degree and Location(s) of Contracture

Patients with disease affecting multiple digits and multiple joints may be more likely to desire amputation. A higher degree of joint contracture, particularly greater than 90 degrees, increases risk of impairment. Patient functional limitations increase significantly as the number of joints, digits, and degrees of contracture increase, increasing the appeal of the option for amputation.

11.3.6 PIP Joint Involvement

The involvement of the PIP joint makes Dupuytren's disease particularly difficult to treat. As evidenced by neurovascular concerns and the risk of autofusion with prolonged disease outlined above, PIP joint contractures are more resistant to treatment than contractures at other joints and are prone to recurrent deformity [8]. The outcomes following surgery for PIP joint contractures are highly variable [3].

11.3.7 Soft Tissue Compromise

Severe disease may compromise the skin and soft tissue of involved digits. Soft tissue compromise may also be worsened by surgical treatment, especially if multiple surgeries are necessary. An assessment of a single surgeon's operative cases for recurrent disease performed at one institution over a 39-year period showed that full-thickness skin grafting was necessary in nearly half of all the patients [9]. If damage to the skin and soft tissue is so extreme that local flaps or skin grafts become impossible, amputation may be necessary.

11.3.8 Other Considerations

Amputation may also be considered if a patient is unwilling or unable to adhere to a postoperative treatment plan and recommended follow-up. Finally, amputation is ideal for patients who desire a rapid recovery.

11.4 Surgical Considerations

When considering surgical options, shared decision-making with the patient is of the utmost importance, particularly in regard to the decision to perform an amputation. When a systematic approach fails to correct flexion contractures, patients should be presented with reasonable alternatives to amputation, such as local flaps, skin grafts, arthroplasty, osteotomy, and arthrodesis [1, 3, 10, 11]. If these alternatives have previously failed, are deemed infeasible, or are refused by the patient, then a thorough assessment of the patient's understanding of the amputation procedure, its risks and benefits, and its potential complications should be conducted. Physicians should ensure that patients understand the finality of amputation and have no reservations about the procedure while assuring the patient's psychological readiness for amputation.

These conversations should also occur before alternative surgical options are attempted, especially for patients with recurrent disease, if amputation is the best or only option after intraoperative evaluation of the anatomical structures and disease severity [5, 11].

When discussing amputation, the surgeon and patient should review the benefits and drawbacks of each level of amputation before making a decision together about which is best for the patient. This involves a comparison of amputation sites at or proximal to the metacarpophalangeal (MCP) joint or distal to it. Ray resection may also be indicated for some patients.

Amputations at or proximal to the MCP joint carry a risk for neuroma and phantom pain, whereas distal amputations have a high risk for recurrent contracture [12]. The risk for recurrence is especially high in disease of the small finger (perhaps because the small finger is the only digit associated with ulnar deep fibrosis), and amputation at or proximal to the MCP joint is recommended for patients with disease of this digit [12]. Alternatively, in disease of the middle finger, amputation at or proximal to the MCP should be avoided if possible [12].

Beyond these considerations, patients and surgeons should decide on amputation levels after considering the specifics of the patient and the concerns and goals of the patient. Patients should be aware that additional amputation could be sought if disease recurs after distal amputation. Similarly, they should be informed that neuropathic pain after digit amputation has been successfully treated with neuromodulators [5]. Finally, minor complaints such as cold intolerance or dysesthesia have been found frequently after all types of amputation and should be mentioned to patients before surgery [12]. Ultimately, there is no clear indication for optimal level of amputation, and a patient-specific decision should be made [5].

Ray resection can be considered. While amputations performed distal to the PIP joint function well without ray resection, those at or proximal to the joint may benefit from improved cosmesis and similar function with concurrent ray resection [13]. In addition to the removal of a cumbersome or painful digit with amputation, ray resection has the advantage of eliminating the gap created by the amputated finger and can produce favorable cosmesis in most cases [13]. Studies have shown that ray resection may lead to a 15–30% decrease in grip and pinch strength [13]. Patients should be made aware of this potential adverse outcome particularly in central digits where ray resection can lead to a gap between digits, malalignment, malrotation or scissoring, decreased dexterity, and unsatisfactory cosmetic outcomes [14, 15]. For central digit ray resection, modern techniques for approximation and soft tissue stabilization should be considered [14, 15].

11.5 Surgical Technique Considerations

Before surgery, physicians and patients should be in full agreement about the choice of amputation as treatment, the level of resection, and whether ray resection will be performed.

Surgery is performed in the preferred setting and sedation level of the patient and surgeon. Standard approach is made for amputation based on the level of resection. Careful attention is paid to designing the incision to ensure appropriate skin flaps for tension-free primary closure. When index ray resection is performed, care is taken to avoid placing the incision in the new first web. The diseased digit is carefully removed.

Careful attention should be given to performing appropriate neurectomy procedures to help reduce the risk of postoperative neuroma pain. Some surgeons advocate for targeted muscle reinnervation (TMR) or regenerative peripheral nerve interface (RPNI), particularly as level of resection moves more proximal. There is no current clear standard of care regarding the use of TMR or RPNI, particularly when performing digital resection distal to the MCP joint. Investigations to establish optimal neurectomy techniques for digit amputation are still ongoing, and surgeons should use their own discretion until additional data is available.

Once resection is complete, it is important to establish supple- and tension-free soft tissue closure. Suture choice should be made based on wound healing potential, patient compliance, patient medical comorbidities, and desire for early aggressive motion with nonabsorbable sutures allowing more reliable healing but requiring postoperative removal. The authors find that postoperative early and aggressive motion, desensitization, and formal hand therapy aid recovery.

11.6 Summary

In the treatment of Dupuytren's contracture, amputation may be beneficial for some patients, especially those with recurrent disease. Surgeons and patients should consider disease severity, functional limitations, and alternative options before making a shared decision about the best treatment plan for each patient. The level of amputation should also be discussed, with the pros and cons of each level weighed against the patient's goals and desired outcomes. For some patients with Dupuytren's disease, amputation is an excellent treatment option that can greatly improve quality of life.

References

1. Tonkin MA, Burke FD, Varian JP. The proximal interphalangeal joint in Dupuytren's disease. J Hand Surg Br. 1985;10(3):358–64. https://doi.org/10.1016/s0266-7681(85)80062-0.
2. Degreef I, De Smet L. Dupuytren's disease: a predominant reason for elective finger amputation in adults. Acta Chir Belg. 2009;109(4):494. https://doi.org/10.1080/00015458.2009.11680467.
3. Wong CR, Huynh MNQ, Fageeh R, McRae MC. Outcomes of management of recurrent Dupuytren contracture: a systematic review and meta-analysis. Hand. 2022;17(6):1104–13. https://doi.org/10.1177/1558944721994220.
4. Alser O, Craig RS, Lane JCE. et al. Serious complications and risk of re-operation after Dupuytren's disease surgery: a population-based cohort study of 121,488 patients in England. Sci Rep. 2020;10:16520. https://doi.org/10.1038/s41598-020-73595-y.
5. Izadpanah A, Rizzo M. Amputation in management of severe Dupuytren's contracture. In: Rizzo M, editor. Dupuytren's contracture. Cham: Springer; 2016. https://doi.org/10.1007/978-3-319-23841-8_17.
6. Denkler K. Surgical complications associated with fasciectomy for dupuytren's disease: a 20-year review of the English literature. Eplasty. 2010;27(10):e15.
7. Andrew JG. Contracture of the proximal interphalangeal joint in Dupuytren's disease. J Hand Surg Br. 1991;16(4):446–8. https://doi.org/10.1016/0266-7681(91)90024-i.
8. Riester S, van Wijnen A, Rizzo M, Kakar S. Pathogenesis and treatment of Dupuytren disease. JBJS Rev. 2014;2(4):e2. https://doi.org/10.2106/JBJS.RVW.M.00072.
9. Hozack BA, Rayan GM. Surgical treatment for recurrent Dupuytren disease. Hand. 2023;18(4):641–7. https://doi.org/10.1177/15589447211060447. Epub 2021 Dec 28
10. Eiriksdottir A, Atroshi I. A new finger-preserving procedure as an alternative to amputation in recurrent severe Dupuytren contracture of the small finger. BMC Musculoskelet Disord. 2019;20(1):323. https://doi.org/10.1186/s12891-019-2701-2.
11. Watson HK, Lovallo JL. Salvage of severe recurrent Dupuytren's contracture of the ring and small fingers. J Hand Surg Am. 1987;12(2):287–9. https://doi.org/10.1016/s0363-5023(87)80291-5.
12. Jensen CM, Haugegaard M, Rasmussen SW. Amputations in the treatment of Dupuytren's disease. J Hand Surg Br. 1993;18(6):781–2. https://doi.org/10.1016/0266-7681(93)90245-b.
13. Blazar PE, Garon MT. Ray resections of the fingers: indications, techniques, and outcomes. J Am Acad Orthop Surg. 2015;23(8):476–84. https://doi.org/10.5435/JAAOS-D-14-00056.
14. O'Brien MS, Singh N. Surgical technique utilizing suture-button device for central metacarpal ray resection. J Hand Surg Am. 2016;41(8):e247–50. https://doi.org/10.1016/j.jhsa.2016.05.005.
15. Mackay B, Wall H, Weaver A, Sexson T, Wall J, Blue M, Doughty M. A novel approach to ray resection of the hand. J Hand Surg Glob Online. 2019;2(1):46–54. https://doi.org/10.1016/j.jhsg.2019.11.001.

Chapter 12
Radiation Therapy in Dupuytren's Disease: Does It Work?

Sasha G. Létourneau and Nina Suh

12.1 Introduction

Although most commonly considered in the treatment of cancers, external beam radiation has been used in the management of numerous benign conditions, including keloid scars, arteriovenous malformations, desmoid tumors, Graves ophthalmopathy, gynecomastia, heterotopic ossification, Dupuytren's disease, plantar fibromatosis (Ledderhose disease) and histiocytosis [1–5]. Radiation therapy is of interest to both clinicians and patients in the context of Dupuytren's disease primarily as a means of controlling early disease to delay invasive treatment [6]. The earliest account of the use of radiation as a treatment for Dupuytren's disease dates back to 1902 as reported by Antoine Béclère [7]. In 1948, Skoog and Slanina, independently reported their findings of the efficacy of radiotherapy in treating Dupuytren's disease [8]. Since this time, numerous studies have emerged investigating the effectiveness of radiotherapy for treating Dupuytren's disease, with most originating in Germany where radiotherapy for Dupuytren's disease is more commonly used than in the rest of the world [4, 7, 9, 10]. This chapter aims to summarize:

1. The rationale for the use of radiation therapy in the treatment of Dupuytren's disease.
2. The evidence behind the effectiveness of radiation therapy in Dupuytren's disease.

S. G. Létourneau
Division of Plastic and Reconstructive Surgery, Western University, London, ON, Canada
e-mail: sletourneau@qmed.ca

N. Suh (✉)
Department of Orthopaedic Surgery, Emory University, Atlanta, GA, USA
e-mail: nina.suh@emory.edu

M. B. Gottschalk et al. (eds.), *Dupuytren's Disease*,
https://doi.org/10.1007/978-3-031-85873-4_12

3. The risks associated with radiation therapy in Dupuytren's disease.
4. The future directions for study in radiation therapy.

12.2 Radiobiological Rationale

Dupuytren's disease has been described histologically in 3 stages of development within the palmar fascia: the proliferative phase, the involutional phase, and the residual phase [11]. In the proliferative stage, fibroblasts proliferate irregularly without any apparent arrangement or structural alignment along usual lines of tension or stress [11]. These proliferating and randomly arranged fibroblasts and myofibroblasts form palpable nodules within the palmar fascia [11, 12]. The involutional stage is characterized by alignment of the fibroblasts within the nodule along lines of stress or tension in the palm, usually the longitudinal axis of the hand [12]. Fibroblast and myofibroblast maturation occurs during this phase, resulting in increasing collagen content within the nodules and decreasing cellularity and vascularity [11]. As a result, the nodules contract, becoming small in diameter and more ill-defined [11, 12]. Meanwhile, the tension placed on the palmar fascia results in functional hypertrophy of the palm's normal fascial bands, forming a reactive fibrous cord proximal to the nodule causing the contracture [11]. In the residual phase, the nodule disappears completely, leaving behind the relatively acellular, tendon-like fibrous cord [11, 12]. Clinically, Dupuytren's disease can generally be observed as a progression from nodules to cords; however, progression occurs at a variable and often unpredictable rate and does not occur at the same rate or extent in all patients [13].

Ionizing radiation targets rapidly proliferating cells directly through damage to DNA as well as indirectly through the formation of reactive oxygen species, which, in turn, disrupts the DNA structure [14]. The result of this damage is an alteration or complete arrest of the cell cycle or cell death [14]. In addition to direct effects on target cells, radiotherapy is also believed to cause indirect effects through, for example, alterations in cell-cell communication and modulation of immune activity [14]. It follows that Dupuytren's disease is most susceptible to radiation in its early phases when nodules are actively developing through rapid hyperproliferation of fibroblasts and myofibroblasts [14]. Meanwhile, in the later phases of disease, fewer target cells remain, and, as a result, the hypocellular and avascular fibrous cords are less radiosensitive [14].

12.3 Radiotherapy Technique

External beam radiation, a form of radiotherapy in which the radiation beam is directed at the body from an external source, is the most commonly used form of radiation in the treatment of Dupuytren's disease [7]. In comparison, brachytherapy providing radiation via implants close to the pathologic tissue has only been used in a minority of studies in small samples [15, 16]. External beam radiation may be delivered through soft (also known as superficial) X-rays (50-kV photons at 25 mA, 15 cm from the skin) or orthovoltage X-rays (120 kV at 20 mA, 40 centimeters from the skin) [7, 17]. Alternately, external radiation may also be delivered using high-speed electrons [7, 18]. The target volume, which is the area of tissue to be irradiated, should include all clinically detectable nodules and cords as well as a safety margin, or surrounding zone of healthy tissue, of at least 0.5–2 centimeters [7, 17]. The remaining uninvolved tissue of the hand is protected from radiation using a rubber lead shield [7, 17, 19].

The dose of radiation, expressed in Gray (Gy), refers to the amount of energy (in Joules) absorbed by one kilogram of tissue [20]. In contrast to the high doses of radiotherapy used in the treatment of cancer, doses of ionizing radiation used to treat Dupuytren's disease and other benign conditions are in the "intermediate" range (20–40 Gy) [2, 4, 17]. The German Society of Radiation Oncology DEGRO guidelines recommend a total dose of 30 Gy or 21 Gy for the treatment of Dupuytren's disease, which corresponds to the dose utilized in most studies (Table 12.1) [17]. The total dose in a course of treatment is delivered in a series of daily treatments ("fractions") [20]. A 30 Gy dose is typically delivered in 5 fractions of 3 Gy applied over 2 series of treatment courses separated by an interval of 6–12 weeks [17, 21]. Alternately, the 21 Gy dose is typically administered in a single series of 7 fractions of 3 Gy [21]. A randomized controlled trial comparing groups receiving the 21 Gy and 30 Gy doses found that progression rates (22% versus 16%, respectively) suggested a non-statistically significant trend in favor of the 30 Gy group being more effective [19].

12.4 Effectiveness of Radiotherapy in Treating Dupuytren's Disease

The literature on this topic is not comprehensive and predominantly originates from Germany, where radiotherapy is more commonly used in the treatment of benign diseases relative to the rest of the world [5, 10]. Twenty-one primary published studies dating back to 1953 were identified as investigating the effectiveness of radiotherapy in Dupuytren's disease (Table 12.1). All but one of these studies are case series with the majority being retrospective. Fourteen of these studies were carried out in Germany and the studies' sample sizes vary considerably from 4 to 718 hands [18, 19]. Additionally, varying classification systems are used to distinguish patients with early and advanced disease, including the Shaw staging system [8, 22], the Iselin staging system [23–26], and the Tubiana et al. staging system or modifications thereof [16, 18, 19, 27–31] (Table 12.2).

Table 12.1 Summary of published studies reporting results of radiation therapy in the management of Dupuytren's disease

Study (year)	Total cohort (hands)	Article type	Classification of disease stage	RT regimen	Dose	Adjunct therapies	Follow-up	Clinical outcome: Regressed/improved	Clinical outcome: Stable	Clinical outcome: Progressed/deteriorated	Salvage procedures reported (n patients)
Randomized clinical trials											
Seegenschmiedt et al. [28]	198 (95 at 30 Gy; 103 at 21 Gy)	Randomized clinical study (published preliminary results)	Tubiana et al. stage ≤ II	5 × 3 Gy over 2 series 8 weeks apart vs. 7 × 3 Gy in 1 series	30 Gy (95 hands) 21 Gy (103 hands)	History of treatment with local excision/partial fasciectomy (25), steroid injection (6), NSAIDs (13), vitamin E (25), other drugs (15), unspecified (12)	>1 year in all patients	**Total**: 54.5% **30 Gy:** 55.8% **21 Gy:** 53.4%	**Total**: 37.4% **30 Gy:** 36.8% **21 Gy:** 37.9%	**Total**: 8.1% **30 Gy:** 7.4% **21 Gy:** 8.7%	Surgery (4)
Seegenschmiedt et al. [19]	718 (293 at 21 Gy; 303 at 30 Gy); 122 control	Randomized controlled trial	21Gy/30Gy: [1]N: 195/199 N/I: 50/53 I: 43/47 II-IV: 5/4	5 × 3 Gy over 2 series 10–12 weeks apart; or 7 × 3 Gy in 1 series	30 Gy vs. 21 Gy	History of treatment with local excision/partial fasciectomy (65), steroid injection (36), NSAIDs (28), vitamin E (45), other drugs (14), unspecified (16)	Median 104 months, range 61–163 months	Not reported	Not reported	21Gy/30Gy/all treated N: 7/3.5/5.3% N/I: 42/30/35.9% I: 58/49/53.3% II-IV: 80/75/77.8% Total: 22/16/18.9% Extension deficit increased in 5.7%	Surgery (21 Gy: 35; 30 Gy: 25) Salvage RT (5.7%)
Retrospective case series											
Finney [8]	25	Case series	[2]Stage 1: 3 Stage 2: 4 Stage 3: 18	3000 r Ra-Moulage	3000r	None	2 to 10 years	Overall: 75% Stage 1: 100% Stage 2: 75% Stage 3: 72%	Overall: 25% Stage 1: 0% Stage 2: 25% Stage 3: 28%	None	Unknown

Finney [22]	43: 25 gamma-radiation (presented in 1953 article); 18 x-radiation	Case series	In X-radiation group: [2]Stage 1: 3 Stage 2: 0 Stage 3: 13 Stage 4: 2	1–3 x 1000 r Ra-Moulage	1500–3000r	None	>18 months	X-radiation group only: 77.8% Stage 1: 100% Stage 2: n/a Stage 3: 76.9% Stage 4: 50.0%	X-radiation group only: 22.2% Stage 1: 0 Stage 2: n/a Stage 3: 23.1% Stage 4: 50.0%	None	Unknown
Wasserburger [33]	146 patients	Case series	*I: 69 II: 46 III: 31	1–3 × 1.000 r Ra-Moulage	1.000–3.000 rad	None	2 to 19 years	"Cured" Overall: 69.8% I: 89.8% II: 56.5% III: 32.2%	Unknown	Unknown	Surgical Intervention (8)
Corsi [15]	13	Case series	"All… in the early stages of the disease"[3]	600–800 r of penetrating radiotherapy then 2200–2500 r of **plesiotherapy**	Variable	Vitamin E	6 months to 3 years	77%	23%	0	Surgical referral (1)
Lukacs et al. [5]	36	Case series	*stage 1: 32 Stage 2: 4	(2 ×4 Gy) × 4 every 2 months	24–40 Gy	None	≤5 years	Stage 1: 81% Stage 2: 75% Total: 81%	Stage 1: 19% Stage 2: 25% Total: 19%	None	Surgical referral (3)
Vogt and Hoschau [25]	109 patients	Case series	[3]I: 98 II: 4 III/IV: 7	(2 × 4 Gy) × 4 every 2 months	32 Gy	None	>3 years	1:21% II: 25% III/IV: - Total: 20%	1:74% II: 50% III/V: 86% Total: 74%	1: 4% II: 25% III/IV: 14% Total: 6%	Unknown

(continued)

Table 12.1 (continued)

Study (year)	Total cohort (hands)	Article type	Classification of disease stage	RT regimen	Dose	Adjunct therapies	Follow-up	Clinical outcome			Salvage procedures reported (n patients)
								Regressed/ improved	Stable	Progressed/ deteriorated	
Iselin and Iselin [26]	46 patients	Case series	All stage I*	(2 × 4 Gy) × 5 every 3 months	40 Gy	None	1–9 years	Total: 52%	Total: 41%	Total: 7%	Unknown
Köhler [24]	33	Case series	All stage I[3]	10 × 2 Gy 3–5 ×/week	20 Gy	None	1–3 years	Total: 21%	Total: 61%	Total: 18%	Surgical intervention (3), salvage RT (3)
Iselin and Iselin [26]	33 patients	Case series	Unknown	5 × 3Gy over 2 series 4–12 weeks apart	9–42 Gy	None	>1.5 years	None	Total: 98%	Total 2%	Unknown
Weinzierl et al. [23]	34 patients	Case series	All stage I[3]	5 × 3 Gy over 2 series 6 weeks apart	15–33 Gy	None	Mean 7 years	9%	41%	50%	Surgery (4)
Keilholz et al. [27]	142 (57 with >5-year follow-up)	Case series	Total/5-year [1]N: 82/28 N/I: 17 /10 I: 30/17 II: 12/1 III: 1/1	5 × 3 Gy over 2 series 6 weeks apart	30 Gy	None	Median 6 years, range 1–12 years	3-mo: 7% N: 2% N/I: 29% I: 10% II/III: 0% 5-year: 11%	3-mo: 92% N: 98% N/I: 71% I: 83%% II/III: 100% 5-year: 67%	3-mo: 1% N: 0% N/I: 0% I: 6.7% II/III: 0% 5-year: 23%	Surgery (6), none in 5-year f/u group
Adamietz et al. [29]	176	Case series	0: 5 [1]N: 76 N/I: 15 I: 65 II: 12 III: 3	5 × 3 Gy Over 2 series 6–8 weeks apart	30 Gy	None	Median 10 years, range 7–18 years	N: 15% I: 6% II: 0% III: 0% Total: 10%	N: 66% I: 29% II: 17% III: 0% Total: 49%	(in + out of field) N: 19% I: 65% II: 83% III: 100% Total: 41%	Surgery (4), salvage RT (10)

Betz et al. [30]	208	Case series	[1]N: 115 N/I: 33 I: 50 II: 7 III: 2 IV: 1	5 × 3 Gy over 2 series 6–8 weeks apart	30 Gy	Prior treatments with recurrence leading to RTX referral: Surgery (8), steroid injection (1)	Median 13 years, range 2–25 years	N: 6% N/I: 30% I: 6% II: 0% III: 0% IV: 0% Total: 10%	N: 81% N/I: 40% I:32% II: 14% III: 0% IV: 0% Total: 59%	(in + out of field) N: 13% N/I: 30% I: 62% II: 86% III: 100% IV: 100% Total: 31%	Surgery (39 patients, 42 cases)
Grenfell and Borg [18]	4	Case series	[1]N: 2 I: 2	5 × 3 Gy over 2 series 6 weeks apart	30Gy	None	Median 35 months, range 34–42 months	100%	–	–	Not mentioned
Latusek et al. [32]	117 patients (number of hands unknown)	Case series	"In the early stages of DD" 61.5% had contractures.	7 × 3 Gy in 1 series	21 Gy	Prior treatment with laser therapy (1%), surgery (13%), ultrasound (1%), local steroid injection (1%)	Mean 4.8 (SD ± 6.11) months, range 1–34 months	57.5%	35%	7.5%	Not mentioned
Banks et al. [48]	8 (11 feet)	Case series	Not reported	5–6 × 3Gy over 2 series 3 months apart	30–36 Gy	None	Mean 12.1 months, range 0.9–30.5 months	71% (but not distinguished from plantar lesions)	24% (but not distinguished from plantar lesions)	5% (but not distinguished from plantar lesions)	Not during study period
Ciernik et al. [16]	6	Case series	[1]I: 2 III: 1 IV: 2	**Brachy-therapy**: 20 Gy in ten fractions after aponeu-rectomy	20 Gy	Palmar aponeurectomy	Mean 14.1 months, range 6–30 months	100%	0	0	Not during study period

(continued)

Table 12.1 (continued)

Study (year)	Total cohort (hands)	Article type	Classification of disease stage	RT regimen	Dose	Adjunct therapies	Follow-up	Clinical outcome			Salvage procedures reported (n patients)
								Regressed/ improved	Stable	Progressed/ deteriorated	
Patient survey studies											
Zirbs et al. [34]	297	Survey study, case series	Symptom duration: <20 months: 56 >20 months: 61	2 × 4 Gy over 4 series 8 weeks apart	32 Gy	Prior treatment with surgery (18), needle fasciotomy (8), local steroid (3), oral vitamins (1), homeopathic cream and massage (1), shock-wave therapy (1), magnetic field therapy (1), NSAIDS (1), hand gymnastics (1), other injections (1)	Median 40 months, range 6–115 months	45% by patient report 21.6% of nodes (regression of 92/426 nodes)	35% by patient report	–	Not mentioned
Schuster et al. [31]	51 sites in the hand (15 sites in the foot)	Pros-pective survey study, case series	[1]N or N/I	7 × 3 Gy in 1 series or 5 × 3 Gy over 2 series 6–8 weeks apart	21 Gy or 30 Gy	Prior treatment with surgery (4), steroid injections (2)	Median 31 months, range 1–61 months	–	–	In-field: 30% In- field after re-irradiation: 21%	Surgery (2); collagenase (1); needle aponeurotomy (2), re-irradiation (4), massage (1)

1. Tubiana et al. classification or a modified version thereof
2. Modification of the Shaw et al. (1951) classification system
3. Iselin classification system
*Staging system unknown or not defined

Table 12.2 Table demonstrating the Shaw staging system [8, 22] the Iselin staging system [26] and the Tubiana staging system modified by Keilholz et al. [27] for Dupuytren's Disease

	Classification systems		
	Shaw (1951)	Iselin (1967)	Tubiana (1966) with modifications (1996)
Grade/stage	1a: Nodule in palmar fascia but not including the skin without finger contracture 1b: Nodule in the skin but not involving the palmar fascia and no finger contracture	0: Small subcutaneous nodules without contracture	N: Nodules, cords or skin retraction in palmar fascia without finger contracture *N/I: Nodules, cords or skin retraction with extension deficit of 1° to 5°
	2: Nodule in fascia involving skin without finger contracture	1: Nodules or cords in palm or up to proximal phalanx with MCPJ contracture	I: Nodules, cords or skin retraction with extension deficit of 6° to 45°
	3: Nodule in fascia involving skin with finger contracture	2: Nodules or cords extend up to the middle phalanx with MCPJ and PIPJ contracture	II: Nodules, cords or skin retraction with extension deficit of 46° to 90°
	4: All 3 prior stages with secondary changes to tendons/joints	3: Nodules or cords extend to the distal phalanx and contracture involving all three phalanges	III: Nodules, cords or skin retraction with extension deficit of 91° to 135°
		4: Severe contracture of the PIPJ resulting in hyperextension at the DIPJ (boutonniere deformity)	III: Nodules, cords or skin retraction with extension deficit >135°

*Keilholz et al. [27] modified the Tubiana classification system to include an N/I intermediate stage with contracture from 1° to 5°
MCPJ metacarpophalangeal joint, *PIPJ* proximal interphalangeal joint, *IPJ* interphalangeal joint

12.4.1 Effectiveness in Early Disease

Despite the lack of comprehensive data on this topic, trends emerging from existing studies over the past 70 years reflect the stage-dependent effectiveness of radiotherapy in Dupuytren's disease, with greater effect occurring at earlier stages of disease. As early as 1953, Finney noted that most patients in their study who achieved full recovery had Shaw stage 1–2 disease [8]. The observation that radiotherapy is more effective in earlier stages of Dupuytren's disease is borne out in subsequent case series, both in short-term and long-term follow-up studies (Table 12.1).

Three early studies of radiotherapy in Dupuytren's disease carried out by Lukacs et al. (1978), Vogt and Hoschau (1980), and Keilholz et al. (1996) classify their outcomes by disease stage, allowing distinction between subgroups of patients at different disease severity [5, 25, 27]. At 5-year follow-up or less, all three studies demonstrate that a higher proportion of early-stage hands achieved improvement or stability of symptoms after radiotherapy compared to hands with later stages of disease (Table 12.1) [5, 25, 27]. Numerous subsequent studies with short- to intermediate-term clinical follow-up—generally considered less than 5 years—included only patients with early-stage disease. For example, in three studies that included only hands with early disease, a majority of participants' hands remained stable or improved at final follow-up [18, 31, 32]. Additionally, the early published results of Seegenschmiedt's randomized clinical trial comparing 21 and 30Gy doses demonstrate that just over half of hands with Tubiana et al. stage II or lower disease had improved and another 37% were stable past one-year follow-up [28].

Similarly, studies with longer-term follow-up demonstrate not only the stage-dependent effect of radiotherapy in Dupuytren's disease but also that effects appear to be maintained as long as 10 years after radiotherapy. Wasserburger et al. (1956) characterize radiotherapy as a "long-term cure" for Dupuytren's disease, reporting cure rates of 90% and 57% in patients with Stage 1 and 2 respectively [33]. More recently, Adamietz et al. (2001) which followed patients for a median of 10 years and Betz et al. (2010) which followed up at a median of 13 years both demonstrate that a smaller proportion of early-stage hands had progressed at final follow-up compared to later stage hands [29, 30].

Finally, although not published in a peer-reviewed journal, Seegenschmiedt et al. (2012) performed the only randomized controlled trial to investigate the effectiveness of radiotherapy in Dupuytren's disease, including both short- and long-term follow-up with stratification of outcomes by disease stage [19]. With a median follow-up interval of 8.7 years, disease progression was seen in only 5% of patients with modified Tubiana et al. N-stage and 36% of patients with N/I-stage disease compared to 34% and 67% respectively in the untreated group [19]. This result is significant in that it shows that patients at all stages of disease experience disease progression and that radiotherapy appears to reduce the rate of progression [19].

12.4.2 Effectiveness in Late Disease

The literature reporting on the effectiveness of radiotherapy in late-stage Dupuytren's disease is scarce. Finney et al. (1955) include a majority of Shaw stage 3–4 patients in both their gamma-ray and x-ray case series, with 28% of these showing no improvement in the gamma-ray series and 27% showing no improvement in the x-ray series [22]. They note that, in these cases, "scar tissue had already been laid down and… would only respond to a limited degree." [8] Another early study, Wasserburger et al. (1956), included a sample in which 21% of patients had stage III disease [33]. They found only 32% regression in the stage III group compared to 57% and 90% in the stage II and stage I groups respectively at "long-term" follow-up [33]. Likely as a result of pathologic evidence that cords lack radiosensitive cells, subsequent studies stratifying outcomes by disease stage include a diminutive minority of patients with late-stage disease (Table 12.1) [5, 19, 27, 29, 30]. Nevertheless, there appears to be a trend, including in the randomized controlled trial, toward lower rates of disease regression and higher rates of disease stability or progression in patients with more advanced Dupuytren's disease, both in short-term and longer-term follow-up studies [5, 19, 27, 29, 30].

12.4.3 Patient-Reported Outcomes

While the literature concerning patient satisfaction with radiation therapy is limited, six studies reporting patient-reported outcomes demonstrate high levels of satisfaction with both the therapy itself and their subjective improvement of symptoms (Table 12.3). Patients' overall satisfaction with the outcome of radiotherapy has been reported at 50–94% [19, 27, 31]. One study used a 10-point scale from "Disappointed" at the low end to "Very satisfied" at the high end and reported an average score of 7.9 (median 9) [34]. Subjective regression of symptoms varied as well across studies from 24% to 66% [19, 28, 30, 34]. Specific symptoms that improved with radiotherapy include burning/itching (27–81%) [30, 31], pain with straining (81%) [31], dysesthesia (4%) [30], and pressure/tension (35–95%) [30, 31].

12.4.4 Need for Salvage Procedures

Need for additional or salvage procedures was reported in half of the included studies; however, of the studies which reported this, only a minority of patients required salvage procedures (Table 12.1). When additional procedures were required, surgical intervention was the most commonly reported additional intervention performed [5, 15, 19, 23, 24, 27–31, 33]. Four studies reported repeat irradiation, with 4 of 6 re-irradiated sites achieving control in one study [19, 24, 29, 31]. Other additional salvage procedures included needle aponeurotomy, collagenase injection, and massage [31].

12.4.5 Comparison with the Natural Progression of Dupuytren's Disease

A criticism of studies investigating radiotherapy in Dupuytren's disease has traditionally been the lack of comparison to control patients, particularly given the rate of progression of Dupuytren's disease can be variable and unpredictable, even in untreated patients [13, 35–38]. The literature on the natural evolution of Dupuytren's disease is limited and further constrained given studies are observational and heterogeneous in terms of design, follow-up, and reporting of both stage and progression. Most studies indicate a clinical disease progression rate of approximately 50%

Table 12.3 Summary of studies reporting patient-reported outcomes after radiation therapy for Dupuytren's disease

Study (year)	Article type	Patients (n)	Total cohort (hands)	Dose	Follow-up	Patient-reported outcome
Keilholz et al. [27]	Retrospective case series	96	142 (57 with >5-year follow-up)	5 × 3 Gy over 2 series 6 weeks apart	Median 6 years, 1–12 years	87% satisfied with long-term outcome
Seegenschmiedt et al. [28]	Randomized clinical study	129 (63 at 30 Gy; 66 at 21 Gy)	198 (95 at 30 Gy; 103 at 21 Gy);	5 × 3 Gy over 2 series 8 weeks apart vs. 7 × 3 Gy in 1 series	>1 year in all patients	At 12-month follow-up: 59% of patients: Regression of symptoms 62% of sites: Regressed by <25% 31% of sites: Regressed by 25–50% 6% of sites: Regressed by 51–75% 2% of sites: Regressed by >75% 36% of patients: Stable symptoms 5% of patients: Progression of symptoms
Betz et al. [30]	Retrospective case series	135	208	5 × 3 Gy over 2 series 6–8 weeks apart	Median 13 years, range 2–25 years	66% reported partial or complete symptom relief (vs. 20% progression): Dysesthesia: 4% relief/2% progression Burning/itching: 27% relief/8% progression Pressure/tension 35% relief/9% progression
Seegenschmiedt et al. [19]	Randomized controlled trial	489 (199 at 21 Gy, 207 at 30 Gy; 83 controls)	718 (293 at 21 Gy; 303 at 30 Gy; 122 control)	5 × 3 Gy over 2 series 10–12 weeks apart; or 7 × 3 Gy in 1 series	Median 104 months, range 61–163 months	50% satisfaction with disease status in treatment groups at last follow-up 48% in 21 Gy 51% in 30 Gy 24% symptom relief in treatment groups at last follow-up 21% in 21 Gy 26% in 30 Gy
Zirbs et al. [34]	Survey study, case series	206	297	2 × 4 Gy over 4 series 8 weeks apart	Median 40 months, range 6–115 months	45%: Regression of symptoms 80%: No further progression (includes regression) Satisfaction on a 10-point Likert scale from "disappointed" to "very satisfied": Average: 7.9/10. Median: 9/10.
Schuster et al. [31]	Prospective survey study, case series	33	51 sites in the hand (15 sites in the foot)	7 × 3 Gy in 1 series or 5 × 3 Gy over 2 series 6–8 weeks apart	Median 31 months, range 1–61 months	94% satisfied 81%: Improved pain with strain 81%: Relieved itch/burn 95%: Improved or stable site pressure. 64%: Improved or stable mobility.

at around 10 years [13, 35, 37]. One study in the Netherlands, however, reported a progression rate of 21.5% at 7 years [36]. By comparison, rates of regression are lower. One study reports a 12% regression rate over an 18-year period [37], while other studies describe rates of 6.5–13% over 5–7 years [36, 38]. Furthermore, correlation between progression and disease stage is contradictory. While one study found significant differences in progression rates across stages at seven-year follow-up [36], another study found no correlation between these two variables at five-year follow-up [38]. The randomized controlled trial carried out by Seegenschmiedt et al. (2012) demonstrates a similar rate of progression in their untreated control group, with 52% progressing over a median interval of 8.7 years [19]. Further, although the sample was biased toward patients at lower stages of disease, rates of progression appeared to escalate with increasing stage. In comparison to both the literature and the study's control group, patients in the 21 Gy and the 30 Gy dose groups experienced significantly lower rates of progression at 22% and 16%, respectively [19].

12.5 Safety

A primary concern with regard to the use of radiation therapy in benign disease is the risk of potential adverse side effects, particularly cancer, outweighing the clinical benefit of treatment. Reported side effects are summarized in Table 12.4.

12.5.1 Acute Side Effects

The definition of "acute" was variable and inconsistently reported in the literature; however, it was typically used to refer to the period within 4–6 weeks of radiotherapy [19, 28, 34]. The overall incidence of acute side effects of any kind was only reported in two studies at 28–39% [19, 31]. In the randomized controlled trial comparing doses of irradiation, side effects were observed to occur more frequently and more intensely after 7 fractions of 3 Gy in the 21 Gy dose group compared to after each of the two series of 5 fractions of 3 Gy in the 30 Gy dose group [19].

12.5.1.1 Dry Skin, Erythema, and Desquamation

Most studies report some degree of mild acute skin reaction involving some combination of dryness, erythema and desquamation or flaking [18, 19, 27, 28, 31, 34]. Rates of these combined symptoms varied in the acute setting from 25% to 43% [19, 27, 28]. Erythema alone was observed in 6–20% [28, 31, 34], with some studies specifying rates of extensive erythema at 2–6% [19, 28]. Dryness was another common side effect, occurring independently in 13–40% of irradiated hands [31, 34].

Table 12.4 Studies reporting acute and long-term side effects after radiation therapy for Dupuytren's disease

Study (year)	Cohort size (hands)	Dose	Follow-up	Side effects
Finney [8]	25	3000 r Ra- Moulage	2–10 years	Slight erythema and skin dryness (n = unknown)
Finney [22]	43 (gamma-ray: 25; medium voltage X-ray: 18)	1–3 × 1000 r Ra-Moulage	>18 months	**Gamma-ray applicator group**: Skin dryness (n = unknown). Immediate paresthesias (n = unknown). **Medium voltage X-ray group:** **Acute**:** Paresthesias (n = unknown). **Long-term:**** Persistent paresthesia (11.1%).
Corsi [15]	13	600–800 r of penetrating radiotherapy then 2200–2500 r of plesiotherapy	6 months to 3 years	Temporary skin rash and epidermolysis (n = unknown).
Weinzierl et al. [23]	34 patients	5 × 3 Gy over 2 series 6 weeks apart	Mean 7 years	Dryness and flaking (32%).
Keilholz et al. [27]	142 (57 with >5-year follow-up)	5 × 3 Gy over 2 series 6 weeks apart	Median 6 years, range 1–12 years	**Acute**:** Acute mild skin reaction (gr. 1), erythema, dry desquamation (43%). Itching and burning ("most"). Radiodermatitis (gr. 2) with pronounced erythema/ moderate edema (10%). **Long-term:**** (77%) Dry skin and increased desquamation (64%) Mild skin atrophy ± slight fibrosis or telangiectasia (13%)
Adamietz et al. [29]	176	5 × 3 Gy over 2 series 6–8 weeks apart	Median 10 years, range 7–18 years	**After median 10 years:** Anhidrosis with severe scaling (25%). Skin atrophy ± telangiectasia (8.5%).

Seegenschmiedt et al. [27]	198 (95 at 30 Gy; 103 at 21 Gy)	5 × 3 Gy over 2 series 8 weeks apart vs. 7 × 3 Gy in 1 series	>1 year in all patients	**Acute (within 4 weeks):** Redness or dryness (38%). Extensive erythema (6%). Dry (5%) or moist (2%) desquamation. Pronounced swelling (2%). Reactions at RT portal (52% in 21 Gy group; 36% in 30 Gy group). **Chronic (at 3-month follow-up):** Dryness, increased desquamation, mild skin atrophy (13% at 3 months, 5% at 12 months). Alteration of heat and pain sensation (4%).
Betz et al. [30]	208	5 × 3 Gy over 2 series 6–8 weeks apart	Median 13 years, range 2–25 years	**Late effects (at last follow-up):** Overall (32%) Dry skin and increased desquamation (gr. 2) (23%). Skin atrophy ± telangiectasia (7%). Erythema lasting up to 1 year (2%). No chronic gr. 3–4, no cancer.
Seegenschmiedt et al. [19]	718 (293 at 21 Gy; 303 at 30 Gy; 122 control)	5 × 3 Gy over 2 series 10–12 weeks apart; or 7 × 3 Gy in 1 series	Median 104 months, range 61–163 months	**Acute (within 6 weeks)**: 28%. Redness/dryness (25%). Extensive erythema, moist desquamation or pronounced swelling (2%). **Chronic (at last follow-up):** (14%). Dryness (rate unspecified). Increased desquamation or mild skin atrophy (LENT grade 1) (rate unspecified). Alteration of heat and pain sensation (rate unspecified).
Grenfell and Borg [18]	4	5 × 3 Gy over 2 series 6 weeks apart	Median 35 months, range 34–42 months	**Acute**:** Minimal fatigue. Mild local edema/erythema.

(continued)

Table 12.4 (continued)

Zirbs et al. [34]	297	2 × 4 Gy over 4 series 8 weeks apart	Median 40 months, range 6–115 months	**Acute (within 4 weeks)**. Erythema (20.4%). Dryness (39.8%). Desquamation (3.8%). **Chronic (>4 weeks).** Dryness (20%). Skin atrophy (3%). Anhidrosis (4%). Telangiectasia (3%). Desquamation (2%). Sensory effects (2%).
Schuster et al. [31]	51 sites in the hand, (15 sites in the foot); 33 patients	7 × 3 Gy in 1 series or 5 × 3 Gy over 2 series 6–8 weeks apart	Median 31 months, range 1–61 months	**Acute**:** 39%. Erythema (20%). Dryness (13.3%). Dry desquamation (5%). Edema (5%). Tenderness (3.3%). Fatigue (1.7%). **Late**:** 30%. Dryness (25%). Weakness (3.3%). Reduced nail health (3.3%). Hyperpigmentation (3.3%).
Latusek et al. [32]	117 patients (number of hands unknown)	7 × 3 Gy in 1 series	Mean 4.8 (SD ± 6.11) months, range 1–34 months	**At last follow-up:** Erythema (7.5%). Superficial epidermal exfoliation (2.5%). Palmar dryness (2.5%).

**Time interval not defined

Desquamation was observed independently of dryness or erythema at rates of 2–5% [28, 31, 34].

12.5.1.2 Edema

Edema in the acute setting was observed in four studies [18, 19, 27, 28, 31]. Edema alone was reported in only one study at a rate of 5% [31]. Additionally, one study noted "pronounced swelling" in conjunction with extensive erythema or moist desquamation in 2% of patients receiving either 21 or 30 Gy [19, 28].

12.5.1.3 Other

Additional symptoms are also described in various studies, including immediate paresthesias [22], itching and burning during the radiation treatments themselves [27], acute tenderness [31], and fatigue [18, 31].

12.5.2 Long-Term Side Effects

Similar to the acute setting, the timing of late or long-term side effects is poorly defined. In some studies, late side effects were evaluated after a specific follow-up interval [28, 34]; however, in most cases, long-term side effects were evaluated at the latest follow-up assessment, which ranged widely across studies from 1 month to 25 years [19, 29, 30, 32]. Overall rates of side effects at last follow-up also varied widely, from 14% at a median follow-up of 104 months to 32% at a median follow-up of 13 years [19, 30].

12.5.2.1 Dry Skin, Erythema, and Desquamation

Dryness and desquamation were the most common cutaneous late sequelae of radiotherapy, with erythema only reported as a long-term side effect in two studies [30, 32]. Dryness and desquamation were commonly reported together at rates ranging widely from 5% to 64% [27–30]. When these symptoms were reported individually, dryness was the more common symptom, seen alone in 2.5–25% of irradiated hands [31, 32, 34].

12.5.2.2 Skin Atrophy and Telangiectasia

A number of studies report skin atrophy with or without fibrosis or telangiectasia [19, 27–30, 34]. Seegenschmiedt et al. (2001) report dryness, increased desquamation, and skin atrophy together at a rate of 13% at three-month follow-up and 5% at

12-month follow-up in their trial of 198 hands receiving 21 or 30 Gy, suggesting that these symptoms may improve with time [28]. Skin atrophy with or without telangiectasia is reported in three case series of hands receiving a 30 Gy total dose with incidence ranging from 7% to 13% [27, 29, 30]. Meanwhile, in another series at 32 Gy, the rate of skin atrophy and telangiectasia are each reported separately at 3% [34].

12.5.2.3 Anhidrosis

Anhidrosis, or lack of sweating, is reported at rates of 4–25% in two studies of patients irradiated with a 30 Gy total dose [29, 34].

12.5.2.4 Other Reported Long-Term Effects

Other long-term toxicities include hyperpigmentation (3%) [31], reduced nail health (3%) [31], paresthesias [22], and other sensory effects (2–4%) [19, 28, 34].

12.5.3 Risk of Cancer

No studies have demonstrated malignancy related to radiotherapy for Dupuytren's disease. However, accurate prediction of the true incidence of cancer in this population is limited by the lack of studies following patients far beyond 10 years post-radiation [4, 14]. The need for longer-term follow-up is illustrated by a case study of a single patient who developed palmar squamous cell carcinoma approximately 40 years after irradiation of both hands with 25.6 Gy for hyperhidrosis [39]. Despite this, the risk of developing cancer as a result of radiotherapy for Dupuytren's disease is considered very low for two reasons. First, the dose of radiation used to treat Dupuytren's disease is considerably lower than the malignancy-inducing doses used in cancer treatment [2, 40]. Second, the population of patients affected by Dupuytren's disease tends to be older, meaning their lifetime opportunity for developing secondary malignancies as a result of low-dose radiotherapy in Dupuytren's disease is reduced [21]. The International Dupuytren's Society estimates the additional risk of developing lethal skin cancer from radiation therapy in Dupuytren's disease to be 0.02%, which is minute relative to the natural lethal cancer coefficient itself (23.945%) and even compared to its degree of uncertainty (0.261%) [40]. In addition, Jansen et al. (2005) estimate the lifetime risk of lethal cancers from irradiation of heel spurs with a total dose of 12 Gy to be 0.6–0.8 per thousand patients in a 25-year-old, 0.2–0.3 per thousand in a 50-year-old, and 0.07–0.1 per thousand in a 75-year-old [41]. Given the doses of radiation use in Dupuytren's disease are approximately double that of heel spurs, the risk estimate in Dupuytren's disease is likely higher. Indeed, Seegenschmiedt et al. (2012) estimate the risk to be 0.5–1% [19].

12.6 Current Societal Recommendations and Guidelines

Various national guidelines have commented on the use of radiation therapy in the management of Dupuytren's disease. The German DEGRO guideline from 2015 recommends performing radiotherapy in the early stages of disease using a total dose of 21–30 Gy [17]. In a 2015 review of radiotherapy for benign disease, the Royal College of Radiologists in the UK acknowledges the role of radiotherapy in the early stages of Dupuytren's disease and recommends a dose of 30 Gy delivered in two series of 15 Gy over five fractions [21]. The statement specifies, however, that radiation should only be used to treat patients with evidence of disease progression within the last 6–12 months [21]. In contrast, in response to a National Institute for Health and Care Excellence (NICE) guidance report, the British Society for Surgery of the Hand (BSSH) released a statement in 2010 stating they would not advocate for radiotherapy as a treatment modality for Dupuytren's disease [42, 43]. In 2022, Kemler et al. published Dutch guidelines on management of Dupuytren's disease advising restriction of radiotherapy for Dupuytren's disease to clinical trials only [44]. However, these Dutch guidelines do not account for the findings of the 2012 randomized controlled trial by Seegenschmiedt et al. which was published in Eaton's *Dupuytren's and Related Hyperproliferative Disorders* [19, 44].

12.7 Conclusion

Although the evidence for radiotherapy in Dupuytren's disease is primarily comprised of observational studies with heterogenous classification systems, follow-up, and outcomes, Dupuytren's disease appears to be responsive to radiation treatment in the early phases of the disease. As shown directly in the randomized controlled trial by Seegenschmiedt et al. (2012), radiotherapy can reduce the rate of progression relative to an observation approach alone [19]. Currently, radiotherapy for the treatment of benign diseases, such as Dupuytren's disease, is most commonly used in Germany. Skepticism remains regarding whether the clinical benefit of radiotherapy outweighs its risks [43]. This presents a barrier to the expansion of radiotherapy treatment in other countries. However, relevant studies demonstrate that side effects are generally limited to benign symptoms, with the most common acute and chronic side effects being erythema, dryness, and desquamation. Additionally, studies have shown high patient satisfaction rates with radiotherapy in terms of clinical benefit and symptom relief. In summary, further high-quality, peer-reviewed studies, including randomized controlled trials, are needed to definitively demonstrate the benefit of radiotherapy for patients with early-stage Dupuytren's disease.

12.8 Future Directions

Since August 2018, an Australian group, GenesisCare, has been conducting a randomized controlled trial (DEPART) [45, 46]. DEPART aims to assess the safety and efficacy of radiotherapy patients with Dupuytren's disease after a 30 Gy dose of radiotherapy in comparison to observation. The study is investigating a "preventive group" comprised of patients undergoing either radiation or observation and an "adjuvant group" of patients who are undergoing fasciectomy, collagenase injection, or needle aponeurotomy followed by either radiotherapy or observation [46]. Patients will be followed for five years. In addition, an observational pilot study is underway in the United States investigating patients' self-reported function using the Southampton Dupuytren's Scoring System questionnaire after undergoing contracture release followed by a 30 Gy dose of radiation [47]. Patients will be assessed six weeks post-radiation as well as one and two years following treatment to assess improvement in function scores [47].

References

1. Eng TY, Abugideiri M, Chen TW, Madden N, Morgan T, Tanenbaum D, et al. Radiation therapy for benign disease: arteriovenous malformations, desmoid tumor, dupuytren contracture, graves ophthalmopathy, gynecomastia, heterotopic ossification, histiocytosis. Hematol Oncol Clin North Am. 2020;34(1):205–27. https://doi.org/10.1016/j.hoc.2019.09.005.
2. Taylor RE, Hatfield P, McKeown SR, Prestwich RJD, Shaffer R. Radiotherapy for benign disease: current evidence, benefits and risks. Clin Oncol. 2015;27(8):433–5.
3. Kriz J, Seegenschmiedt HM, Bartels A, Micke O, Muecke R, Schaefer U, et al. Updated strategies in the treatment of benign diseases – a patterns of care study of the german cooperative group on benign diseases. Adv Radiat Oncol. 2018;3(3):240–4. https://doi.org/10.1016/j.adro.2018.02.008.
4. McKeown SR, Hatfield P, Prestwich RJD, Shaffer RE, Taylor RE. Radiotherapy for benign disease; assessing the risk of radiation-induced cancer following exposure to intermediate dose radiation. Br J Radiol. 2015;88(1056):20150405.
5. Lukacs S, Braun-Falco O, Goldschmidt H. Radiotherapy of benign dermatoses: indications, practice, and results. J Dermatol Surg Oncol. 1978;4(8):620–5. https://doi.org/10.1111/j.1524-4725.1978.tb00512.x.
6. Werker PMN, Degreef I. Alternative and adjunctive treatments for Dupuytren disease. Hand Clin. 2018;34(3):367–75. https://doi.org/10.1016/j.hcl.2018.03.005.
7. Eberlein B, Biedermann T. To remember: radiotherapy – a successful treatment for early Dupuytren's disease. J Eur Acad Dermatol Venereol. 2016;30(10):1694–9.
8. Finney R. Dupuytren's contracture a radiotherapeutic approach. Lancet. 1953;262(6795):1064–6.
9. Seegenschmiedt MH, Katalinic A, Makoski HB, Haase W, Gademann G, Hassenstein E. Radiation therapy for benign diseases: patterns of care study in Germany. Int J Radiat Oncol Biol Phys. 2000;47(1):195–202.
10. Fionda B, Lancellotta V, Casà C, Boldrini L, Marazzi F, Cellini F, et al. Radiotherapy for benign disorders: current use in clinical practice. Eur Rev Med Pharmacol Sci. 2021;25(9):3440–3. https://doi.org/10.26355/eurrev_202105_25824.

11. Luck JV. Dupuytren's contracture; a new concept of the pathogenesis correlated with surgical management. J Bone Joint Surg Am. 1959;41-A(4):635–64.
12. Shih B, Bayat A. Scientific understanding and clinical management of Dupuytren disease. Nat Rev Rheumatol. 2010;6(12):715–26.
13. Millesi H, Hueston JT, Tubiana R. The clinical and morphological course of dupuytren's disease. In: Dupuytren's disease. London: Grune & Stratton; 1974. p. 49–60.
14. Rödel F, Fournier C, Wiedemann J, Merz F, Gaipl US, Frey B, et al. Basics of radiation biology when treating hyperproliferative benign diseases. Front Immunol. 2017;8(May)
15. Corsi M. Radiotherapy of Dupuytren's disease. Friuli Med. 1966;21(3):391–403.
16. Ciernik IF, Goldschmidt P, Wösle M, Winter J. Feasibility of aponeurectomy in combination with perioperative 192Ir high dose rate brachytherapy for Dupuytren's disease. Strahlenther Onkol. 2021;197(10):903–8.
17. Seegenschmiedt MH, Micke O, Niewald M, Mücke R, Eich HT, Kriz J, et al. DEGRO guidelines for the radiotherapy of non-malignant disorders: part III: hyperproliferative disorders. Strahlenther Onkol. 2015;191(7):541–8.
18. Grenfell S, Borg M. Radiotherapy in fascial fibromatosis: a case series, literature review and considerations for treatment of early-stage disease. J Med Imaging Radiat Oncol. 2014;58(5):641–7.
19. Seegenschmiedt MH, Keilholz L, Wielpütz M, Schubert C, Fehlauer F. Long-term outcome of radiotherapy for early stage Dupuytren's disease: a phase III clinical study. In: Eaton C, et al., editors. Dupuytren's disease and related hyperproliferative disorders. Berlin: Springer-Verlag; 2012. p. 349–71.
20. Shaffer R. Radiotherapy for Dupuytren's disease. In: Böttcher R, editor. Handchirurgie Weltweit eV. Cologne: GMS; 2016. p. 1–5. https://doi.org/10.5680/lhhs000015.
21. Royal College of Radiologists. A review of the use of radiotherapy in the UK for the treatment of benign clinical conditions and benign tumours. London: The Royal College of Radiologists; 2015.
22. Finney R. Dupuytren's contracture. Br J Radiol. 1955;28(335):610–4.
23. Weinzierl G, Flügel M, Geldmacher J. Lack of effectiveness of alternative non-surgical treatment procedures of Dupuytren contracture. Chir Z Alle Geb Oper Medizen. 1993;64(6):492–4.
24. Köhler AH. Radiotherapy of Dupuytren's contracture. Radiobiol Radiother (Berl). 1984;25(6):851–3.
25. Vogt HJ, Hochschau L. The treatment of Dupuytren's contracture. A social medical problem. Munch Med Wochenschr. 1980;122(4):125–30.
26. Iselin M, Iselin F. Chapitre XXI: Maladie de Dupuytren. In: Tubiana R, editor. Traité de chirurgie de la main. Paris/New York/Barcelone: Éditions Médicales Flammarion; 1967. p. 667–713.
27. Keilholz L, Seegenschmiedt MH, Sauer R. Radiotherapy for prevention of disease progression in early-stage Dupuytren's contracture: initial and long-term results. Int J Radiat Oncol. 1996;36(4):891–7.
28. Seegenschmiedt MH, Olschewski T, Guntrum F. Radiotherapy optimization in early-stage dupuytren's contracture: first results of a randomized clinical study. Int J Radiat Oncol Biol Phys. 2001;49(3):785–98.
29. Adamietz B, Keilholz L, Sauer R. Die radiotherapie des Morbus Dupuytren im fruhstadium. Strahlenther Onkol. 2001;11:604–10.
30. Betz N, Ott OJ, Adamietz B, Sauer R, Fietkau R, Keilholz L. Radiotherapy in early-stage dupuytren's contracture long-term results after 13 years. Strahlenther Onkol. 2010;186(2):82–90.
31. Schuster J, Saraiya S, Tennyson N, Nedelka M, Mukhopadhyay N, Weiss E. Patient-reported outcomes after electron radiation treatment for early-stage palmar and plantar fibromatosis. Pract Radiat Oncol. 2015;5(6):e651–8.
32. Latusek T, Miszczyk L, Gierlach G, Zajac P. An effectiveness evaluation of the palmar fascia irradiation of patients suffering from Dupuytren's disease. Nowotwory. 2017;67(3):162–7.
33. Wasserburger K. Therapy of Dupuytren's contracture. Strahlentherapie. 1956;100(4):546–60.

34. Zirbs M, Anzeneder T, Bruckbauer H, Hofmann H, Brockow K, Ring J, et al. Radiotherapy with soft X-rays in Dupuytren's disease – successful, well-tolerated and satisfying. J Eur Acad Dermatol Venereol. 2015;29(5):904–11.
35. Reilly RM, Stern PJ, Goldfarb CA. A retrospective review of the management of Dupuytren's nodules. J Hand Surg. 2005;30(5):1014–8.
36. Van Den Berge BA, Werker PMN, Broekstra DC. Limited progression of subclinical Dupuytren's disease results from a prospective cohort study. Bone Joint J. 2021;103(4):704–10.
37. Gudmundsson KG, Arngrimsson R, Jónsson T. Eighteen years follow-up study of the clinical manifestations and progression of Dupuytren's disease. Scand J Rheumatol. 2001;30(1):31–4.
38. Broekstra DC, Lanting R, Werker PMN, van den Heuvel ER. Disease course of primary Dupuytren disease: 5-year results of a prospective cohort study. Plast Reconstr Surg. 2022;149(6):1371–8.
39. Campanelli A, Lubbe J. Palmar squamous-cell carcinoma. N Engl J Med. 2019;381(11):1058.
40. Dupuytren. Estimate of the risk of cancer caused by radiation therapy of Dupuytren's Disease. Dupuytren's International Society; 2019.
41. Jansen JTM, Broerse JJ, Zoetelief J, Klein C, Seegenschmiedt MH. Estimation of the carcinogenic risk of radiotherapy of benign diseases from shoulder to heel. Radiother Oncol. 2005;76(3):270–7.
42. Radiation therapy for early Dupuytren's disease. National Institute for Health and Care Excellence (NICE); 2016, p. 1–4. Available from: https://www.nice.org.uk/guidance/ipg573/resources/information-for-the-public-pdf-3539938480837
43. Shewring D. Dupuytren's disease and radiotherapy. Br Soc Surg Hand. 2020:1–9.
44. Kemler MA, de Wijn RS, van Rijssen AL, van Kooij YE, Ottenhof MPM, van Heijl M, et al. Dutch multidisciplinary guideline on Dupuytren disease. J Hand Surg Glob Online. 2022;5:1–6. https://doi.org/10.1016/j.jhsg.2022.11.008.
45. GenesisCare. DEPART; 2021. Available from: https://www.genesiscare.com/au/specialists/research/clinical-trials/depart
46. Jarad Martin. Australian New Zealand Clinical Trials Registry. 2018. Trial Review. Available from: https://www.anzctr.org.au/Trial/Registration/TrialReview.aspx?id=375241
47. Dusenbery K. Clinicaltrials.gov. 2023. Post-contracture release radiation for Dupuytren's disease. Available from: https://clinicaltrials.gov/ct2/show/NCT04122313
48. Banks JS, Wolfson AH, Subhawong TK. T2 signal intensity as an imaging biomarker for patients with superficial fibromatoses of the hands (Dupuytren's disease) and feet (Ledderhose disease) undergoing definitive electron beam irradiation. Skeletal Radiol. 2018;47(2):243–51.

Chapter 13
The Role of Steroids in Dupuytren's Disease Management

Osvaldo Conde Lorenzo, Jeremy E. Raducha, and Christopher Klifto

13.1 Introduction

Dupuytren's disease is a benign condition that affects the hand and can cause significant functional impairment. There are various treatment options typically used to manage the disease, e.g., partial fasciectomy, percutaneous needle aponeurotomy (PNA), and collagenase injections, but all carry a fairly high recurrence rate. Corticosteroid injections are another treatment option which has been described in the literature for decades but is not commonly utilized. The goal of these injections is to slow the disease's development as well as soften and reduce the size of the nodules. However, there is debate about the best administration methods, dose schedules, and overall safety and efficacy of corticosteroid injections in the setting of Dupuytren's disease. By providing a comprehensive review of the current literature about corticosteroid injections in Dupuytren's disease, this chapter seeks to consolidate available information that may prove useful in clinical practice. This chapter will discuss the pathophysiological causes and biochemical foundations of Dupuytren's disease, before considering corticosteroids' mechanisms of action and types of administration. We will then compare and contrast corticosteroid efficacy and safety with the other available treatments.

O. C. Lorenzo
San Juan Bautista School of Medicine, Caguas, Puerto Rico

J. E. Raducha
St Luke's University Health Network, Bethlehem, PA, USA

C. Klifto (✉)
Duke University, Durham, NC, USA
e-mail: christopher.klifto@duke.edu

M. B. Gottschalk et al. (eds.), *Dupuytren's Disease*,
https://doi.org/10.1007/978-3-031-85873-4_13

13.2 Background

13.2.1 Biochemistry of Dupuytren's Disease

Dupuytren's nodules and cords exhibit an increase in the ratio of Type III to Type I collagen, a pattern similar to hypertrophic scar and granulation tissue[1]. Initially, there is fast production of immature collagen, especially Type III collagen, without any indication of collagen fibril contraction. The tissue fabric gradually shortens as a result of the contractile stresses generated by myofibroblasts on one another and the freshly created collagen fibrils, even if the collagen produced is initially of normal length. The formation of Dupuytren's contracture is thought to be aided by these myofibroblasts and the actin molecules within. The overexpression of prostaglandins, lysophosphatidic acid (LPA), and platelet-derived growth factor (PDGF) also contributes to the promotion of myofibroblast contracture. Interleukin 1 alpha and beta, transforming growth factor beta (TGF-beta), and basic fibroblast growth factor (bFGF) are also linked to signaling and proliferation in the illness. These biochemical elements allow Dupuytren's disease to develop and advance, further emphasizing the intricacy of its underlying processes.

The process is eventually stabilized when myofibroblasts vanish and dense collagenous fiber bundles start to grow, separated by classic fibroblasts [2]. Mature Dupuytren's nodules and cords are characterized by larger concentrations of water, collagen, and chondroitin sulfate, along with larger ratios of soluble collagens and reducible cross-links, all of which point to the production of new collagen [3]. Reduced fibrinolytic ability, which permits the accumulation of fibrin in the palmar fascia, is also a significant component of the biochemistry of Dupuytren's disease. The creation and growth of nodules are aided by this deposition as well as the fibroblasts' adherence to polymerizing fibrin.

13.2.2 How Steroids Act as Antifibrotic Agents/Which Steroid to Use?

Dupuytren's nodules and keloid scars are both characterized by an overabundance of collagen synthesis, which results in the creation of aberrant tissue. Triamcinolone acetonide has been used to treat keloid scars by softening the abundant collagen [4], and by extrapolation, it may be beneficial in the treatment of Dupuytren's nodules.

Triamcinolone, which is categorized as a 9-alpha fluor-hydrocortisone, efficiently breaks down insoluble collagen in keloids and hypertrophic scars. Triamcinolone makes insoluble collagen salt-soluble, which makes it easier for the body to absorb and then excrete [5]. The medication accomplishes this by blocking alpha-2 macroglobulin, which raises collagenase activity and encourages the destruction of insoluble collagen [4]. Hydrocortisone, another corticosteroid, on the other hand, transforms insoluble collagen into acid-soluble collagen, which the body does not absorb.

When used within 24 hours following an injury, triamcinolone demonstrates a special capacity to reduce fibroplasia in healing wounds. This characteristic is particularly pertinent to Dupuytren's nodules, which resemble hypertrophic scars and are distinguished by a high collagen concentration and an aberrant ratio of type III to type I collagen [6]. Triamcinolone acetonide has been shown in clinical investigations to significantly soften and flatten hypertrophic scars and keloids after intralesional injection, supporting the drug's therapeutic potential [7].

Case studies have also shown the efficacy of triamcinolone injections and intralesional fenestration in treating Ledderhose nodules in the plantar foot. These patients underwent two injections, which resulted in a notable decrease in discomfort and lesion volume at 12-month follow-up [8].

Fibromatoses, a class of proliferative fibroblastic illnesses, resemble Dupuytren's nodules and keloid scars histologically. Spindle-shaped myofibroblasts, substantial intercellular collagen fibers, compressed and elongated arteries, and various extracellular myxoid matrix appearances are features of these illnesses [9]. Triamcinolone's therapeutic mechanism, which is similar to that of anti-macrophage serum, is further strengthened by its dose-dependent effect on the macrophage-fibroblast-collagen cascade.

Despite the positive results of triamcinolone treatment, reactivation of Dupuytren's nodules can happen in many patients within 1–3 years following the last injection, frequently requiring repeated doses [10]. However, triamcinolone acetonide intralesional injection may have the ability to change the course of the illness. One in vitro study has shown steroids cause apoptosis in cultured Dupuytren's cells but not in palmar fascia or fascia lata cells, indicating a selective impact on the target cells [11].

13.2.3 Technique for Injecting Steroid into Dupuytren's Nodule

According to Ketchum [4], the approach entails a direct intralesional injection. However, due to the density of the tissue, delivering the injection necessitates a large amount of pressure on the syringe.

To reduce motion during the treatment, lidocaine is used near the nodule to anesthetize the area. It should be noted that lidocaine should not be coupled with triamcinolone during injection. This precaution is taken to guarantee that the lidocaine takes action before the steroid injection. Injecting too quickly may cause the patient's hand to move, resulting in an injection into normal tissues rather than the targeted nodule. Furthermore, there is a danger that lidocaine will precipitate triamcinolone, making the steroid less effective [4].

The majority of people require three injections, 6 weeks apart. The dose for smaller nodules is 40–60 mg, while the dosage for bigger nodules is 80–120 mg. Because of transient adrenal suppression, 100 mg is generally the maximum dosage in women [4]. Patients may suffer discomfort for up to 24 hours following the injection. However, the second and third injections become easier to administer as the treatment proceeds since significant alterations in the afflicted tissue have been observed over time.

13.3 When to Use Steroids?

13.3.1 Early Nodules

Dupuytren's begins as nodules which can be tender in the earlier stages before quiescing and potentially growing into chords which tighten and cause contracture across the joints into the fingers [12].

In a study by [10] triamcinolone was administered to 63 patients (75 hands) with Dupuytren's nodules who had less than 15 degrees of metacarpophalangeal (MP) contracture and no proximal interphalangeal (PIP) contracture throughout a four-year period. The dose of Triamcinolone ranged from 60–120 mg each injection, with males commonly receiving 100–120 mg and women receiving less than 80 mg. The injections were given at 6-week intervals for a total of three treatments. If the nodules did not improve after 6 months, the injections were resumed at 6-week intervals. Each nodule got 3.2 shots on average.

Regression of the disease was exhibited in 97% of the treated hands, with nodules softening and flattening. Most hands had a 60–80% reduction in nodule size, with some even seeing total resolution. However, a single injection did not result in considerable improvement. Furthermore, any existing joint contractures were not affected. Within 1–3 years, over half of the patients had a recurrence of the condition, needing another round of injections. There was only one patient who needed surgery. Transient pigmentation or subcutaneous fat shrinkage at the injection site were the most common problems seen, with the majority recovering within 6 months.

Additionally, two incidences of flexor tendon ruptures in golfers were documented, however these happened outside of the research period and included patients who did not follow the 6-month rest period after having more than three injections.

Other research, conducted in Taiwan, looked at 37 patients and 49 hands who received 5 mg triamcinolone acetonide injections for 3 months, revealed no advancement of nodes after a 6-month follow-up, with only 2 patients experiencing reactivation after a 5-year follow-up. The treated Dupuytren nodule diameters decreased by 40% 6 months after injection and 56% at the final follow-up [13].

13.3.2 After Release to Maintain Correction

In a randomized control trial [14], the use of postoperative steroid injections was investigated as a technique to sustain correction following percutaneous needle aponeurotomy (PNA) for Dupuytren's contracture. The experiment included 47 patients undergoing primary PNA who were randomly allocated to one of two groups: one that received no steroids and the other that received injections immediately after PNA, 6 weeks later, and 3 months later. Following release, the injections were given into the thicker remaining cords.

Surprisingly, there was no change in range of motion (ROM) between the two groups at the metacarpophalangeal (MP) joint, while the steroid group had considerably superior ROM at the proximal interphalangeal (PIP) joint. Combining the mechanical effects of PNA with the molecular actions of the corticosteroid Triamcinolone led to a much greater degree of correction than PNA alone [15]. Notably, the study did not analyze post-operative treatment, splint use, or home exercise program adherence, which might be a significant confounding variable influencing the findings. As such, the evaluation of additional variables is required to properly discern the impact of this therapy method in clinical practice.

In a long-term follow-up of post-operative corticosteroid injection (CSI) following percutaneous needle aponeurotomy (PNA) for Dupuytren's contracture, 44 out of 47 patients completed the 53-month follow-up [14]. According to the findings of the study, 62% of patients in the non-injection group and 30% of patients who got triamcinolone injections after PNA needed a second treatment on the same digit(s) (retreatment). This difference in retreatment rates across groups, however, was not determined to be statistically significant. Furthermore, there were no significant changes in the mean time to retreatment or the mean total active extension deficit (TAED) immediately before retreatment between the two groups. These data shed light on the long-term outcomes and retreatment rates following post-operative CSI following PNA.

Oral corticosteroids may also be a supplementary treatment option following collagenase injection. In a study [16] with patients who received oral prednisone following collagenase Clostridium histolyticum (CCH) (10 mg/day for 2 weeks) for Dupuytren's contracture with a 1-year follow-up, the prednisolone group had a noticeably higher mean total active motion (TAM) at days 7 and 30. In the prednisolone group, the mean TAM was 235 degrees at day 7, whereas it was 228 degrees in the control group. At day 30, the mean TAM in the prednisolone group was 241 degrees, while it was 233 degrees in the control group. This suggests that after the CCH was injected, oral prednisolone reduced connective tissue edema.

13.4 Complications

Although corticosteroid injections for Dupuytren's disease are often thought to be safer than other alternative therapies, they also carry the risk of complications. Corticosteroid administration can result in dermal depigmentation, changing the color of the skin and perhaps impairing the treated area's cosmetic appeal. Another consequence might be subcutaneous fat atrophy, which leads to a hollowed-out appearance after frequent corticosteroid injections. These injections, although having a generally safer profile, have been linked to a higher risk of tendon rupture, especially when given deeply into the nodules. Corticosteroid drugs can also cause allergic responses, adding another level of uncertainty to the therapeutic procedure. While the use of corticosteroid injections for the treatment of Dupuytren's disease has benefits in terms of safety, the risks they carry underscore the need for cautious planning and monitoring.

13.5 Comparison to Other Treatments

13.5.1 Collagenase Clostridium Histolyticum Injections

Collagenase Clostridium histolyticum (CCH) injections are another method of treatment for contractures of Dupuytren's disease for patients who do not want to undergo surgical procedures or to avoid the risks and complications from surgery [17].

Its major impact is the disruption of cords via the breakdown of collagen rather than the nodule. However, the cost of using CCH may represent an issue for the patients and it requires a minimum of two visits in a short period of time for treatment [4]. Side effects include localized swelling/ecchymosis, pruritus, and transient lymphadenopathy in the upper extremity. Flexor tendon ruptures have also been reported in the literature. The overall recurrence rates are also high with approximately 20% recurrence rate per year, however there is industry-produced research that shows a lower recurrence rate for the more moderate cords when excluding the rapid recurrences. Collagenase injections treatment results in greater reintervention rates at 2 years when compared to reintervention rates to needle aponeurotomy at 5 years, and the highest cumulative expenses [18].

13.5.2 Percutaneous Needle Aponeurotomy

Percutaneous needle aponeurotomy is a procedure that can be carried out in an office setting with local anesthesia, and it can be repeated on multiple occasions. It provides instant results, quick recovery, and is inexpensive when done in the office

[18]. It also does not exclude future procedures such as fasciectomy. Unfortunately, PNA has high recurrence rates, at about 20% recurrence per year [19].

13.5.3 Partial Fasciectomy

In a partial or limited fasciectomy the majority of the affected nodules are removed, and the neurovascular bundle is traced out. This technique has a lower recurrence rate than the percutaneous options, approximately 5% recurrence per year, however it also causes swelling and stiffness, with a longer recovery [19]. Patients can use finger flexion as a result of stiffness, which can limit function more than their pre-operative loss of extension. Overall, it is an effective procedure for the treatment of contractures of MP and PIP joints of all severities.

13.6 Conclusions

Steroids' therapeutic benefits in the management of Dupuytren's disease go beyond their anti-inflammatory actions and increased collagenase activity. Triamcinolone, a strong corticosteroid, has shown promise as a multimodal treatment that tackles many facets of the disease's etiology.

The affordability of triamcinolone is one of its significant benefits. Traditional Dupuytren's disease treatments, such as surgical excision, can be quite expensive owing to hospital and surgeon costs, and post-operative care. Triamcinolone injections, on the other hand, provide a less expensive outpatient alternative that can potentially lessen the financial strain on both patients and healthcare systems.

Numerous medicinal uses of triamcinolone have given rise to substantial research and well-established documentation of its safety profile. The rare potential side effects/complications are reduced when administered over a strict treatment timeline with an adequate rest period between the third and fourth injection.

Triamcinolone effectively treats the underlying pathology in Dupuytren's disease in addition to relieving symptoms by decreasing inflammatory factors and boosting collagenase activity. Triamcinolone's capacity to postpone recurrence and reduce the growth of nodules may be one of the treatment's most encouraging effects. The necessity for recurrent injections or surgical treatments might be considerably reduced thanks to this preventative element of therapy. This not only improves the therapy's long-term efficacy but also eases the strain on patients who would otherwise need to undergo repeated medical treatments.

The use of triamcinolone as a treatment for Dupuytren's disease takes advantage of its anti-inflammatory qualities, collagenase activity augmentation, cost-effectiveness, safety profile, and potential for recurrence prevention. Triamcinolone offers a promising avenue for both symptomatic treatment and disease modification by focusing on many facets of the illness's pathophysiology. However, more research is needed to better define its role in Dupuytren's disease treatment given its high recurrence rate and the need for multiple injections.

References

1. Brickley-Parsons D, Glimcher MJ, Smith RJ, Albin R, Adams JP. Biochemical changes in the collagen of the palmar fascia in patients with Dupuytren's disease. J Bone Joint Surg Am. 1981;63:787–97.
2. Salamon A, Hámori J. Possible role of myofibroblasts in the pathogenesis of Dupuytren's contracture. Acta Morphol Acad Sci Hung. 1980;28:71–82.
3. Bazin S, Le Lous M, Duance VC, Sims TJ, Bailey AJ, Gabbiani G, D'Andiran G, Pizzolato G, Browski A, Nicoletis C, Delaunay A. Biochemistry and histology of the connective tissue of Dupuytren's disease lesions. Eur J Clin Investig. 1980;10:9–16. https://doi.org/10.1111/j.1365-2362.1980.tb00003.x.
4. Ketchum LD. The rationale for treating the nodule in Dupuytren's disease. Plast Reconstr Surg Glob Open. 2014;2:e278. https://doi.org/10.1097/GOX.0000000000000249.
5. Ketchum LD, Robinson DW, Masters FW. The degradation of mature collagen: a laboratory study. Plast Reconstr Surg. 1967;40:89–91. https://doi.org/10.1097/00006534-196707000-00016.
6. Badalamente MA, Hurst LC. The biochemistry of Dupuytren's disease. Hand Clin. 1999;15:35–42. https://doi.org/10.1016/S0749-0712(21)00437-6.
7. Ketchum LD, Smith J, Robinson DW, Masters FW. The treatment of hypertrophic scar, keloid and scar contracture by triamcinolone acetonide. Plast Reconstr Surg. 1966;38:209–18. https://doi.org/10.1097/00006534-196609000-00005.
8. Flanagan G, Burt N, Reilly IN. Intralesional fenestration and corticosteroid injection for symptomatic Ledderhose disease of the foot: two case reports. SAGE Open Med Case Rep. 2021;9:2050313X211011813. https://doi.org/10.1177/2050313X211011813.
9. Goldblum JR, Folpe AL, Weiss SW. Benign fibroblastic/myofibroblastic proliferations, including superficial fibromatoses – ClinicalKey. In: Enzinger and Weiss's soft tissue tumors. Elsevier Saunders; 2014.
10. Ketchum LD, Donahue TK. The injection of nodules of Dupuytren's disease with triamcinolone acetonide. J Hand Surg. 2000;25:1157–62. https://doi.org/10.1053/jhsu.2000.18493.
11. Meek RMD, McLellan S, Reilly J, Crossan JF. The effect of steroids on Dupuytren's disease: role of programmed cell death. J Hand Surg. 2002;27:270–3. https://doi.org/10.1054/jhsb.2001.0742.
12. Seyhan H, Kopp J, Schultze-Mosgau S, Horch RE. Increased metabolic activity of fibroblasts derived from cords compared with nodule fibroblasts sampling from patients with Dupuytren's contracture. Plast Reconstr Surg. 2006;117:1248–52. https://doi.org/10.1097/01.prs.0000204585.97844.7e.
13. Yin C-Y, Yu H-HM, Wang J-P, Huang Y-C, Huang T-F, Chang M-C. Long-term follow-up of Dupuytren disease after injection of triamcinolone acetonide in Chinese patients in Taiwan. J Hand Surg Eur. 2017;42:678–82. https://doi.org/10.1177/1753193417690961.
14. McMillan C, Binhammer P. Steroid injection and needle aponeurotomy for Dupuytren disease: long-term follow-up of a randomized controlled trial. J Hand Surg. 2014;39:1942–7. https://doi.org/10.1016/j.jhsa.2014.07.018.
15. McMillan C, Binhammer P. Steroid injection and needle aponeurotomy for Dupuytren contracture: a randomized, controlled study. J Hand Surg. 2012;37:1307–12. https://doi.org/10.1016/j.jhsa.2012.04.026.

16. Abe Y. Effect of Oral prednisolone after collagenase injection for Dupuytren's contracture: a randomized, controlled trial with a 1-year follow-up. J Hand Microsurg. 2020;14:113. https://doi.org/10.1055/s-0040-1709097.
17. Malafa MM, Lehrman C, Criley JW, Amirlak B. Collagenase Dupuytren contracture: achieving single treatment success with a hand therapist-based protocol. Plast Reconstr Surg Glob Open. 2016;4:e629. https://doi.org/10.1097/GOX.0000000000000565.
18. Leafblad ND, Wagner E, Wanderman NR, Anderson GR, Visscher SL, Maradit Kremers H, Larson DR, Rizzo M. Outcomes and direct costs of needle aponeurotomy, collagenase injection, and Fasciectomy in the treatment of Dupuytren contracture. J Hand Surg. 2019;44:919–27. https://doi.org/10.1016/j.jhsa.2019.07.017.
19. Denkler KA, Park KM, Alser O. Treatment options for Dupuytren's disease: tips and tricks. Plast Reconstr Surg Glob Open. 2022;10:e4046. https://doi.org/10.1097/GOX.0000000000004046.

Chapter 14
Designing Flaps and Skin Incisions

Spencer B. Chambers

14.1 Introduction

Incision planning is critical for all procedures but is particularly important for hand surgery. The complex motion and sensation that give the hand its utility can be easily hampered by a sensitive scar or contracture. Dupuytren's disease excision requires additional considerations because pathologic changes can distort anatomy displacing critical structures and compromising skin vascularity. Designing the ideal incision requires an understanding of skin flap physiology, wound healing, geometric principles, and expected anatomic aberrations. Although diseased fascia can impact the entire hand, the digits represent a specific challenge due to the density of anatomic structures as well as burden of disease. By applying these principles, secondary complications such as skin flap necrosis, contracture, and wound dehiscence can be avoided while allowing efficient and safe excision of disease.

14.2 Basic Science

There are numerous incision designs for Dupuytren's surgery (Fig. 14.1, Table 14.1) [1–6]. Each has benefits and drawbacks but all rely on basic tenets of hand surgery including an understanding of skin flap physiology, normal healing, and technical execution. When principles are correctly applied, a variety of solutions are possible.

S. B. Chambers (✉)
Department of Plastic & Reconstructive Surgery. Roth|McFarlane Hand & Upper Limb Center, Western University, London, ON, Canada

M. B. Gottschalk et al. (eds.), *Dupuytren's Disease*,
https://doi.org/10.1007/978-3-031-85873-4_14

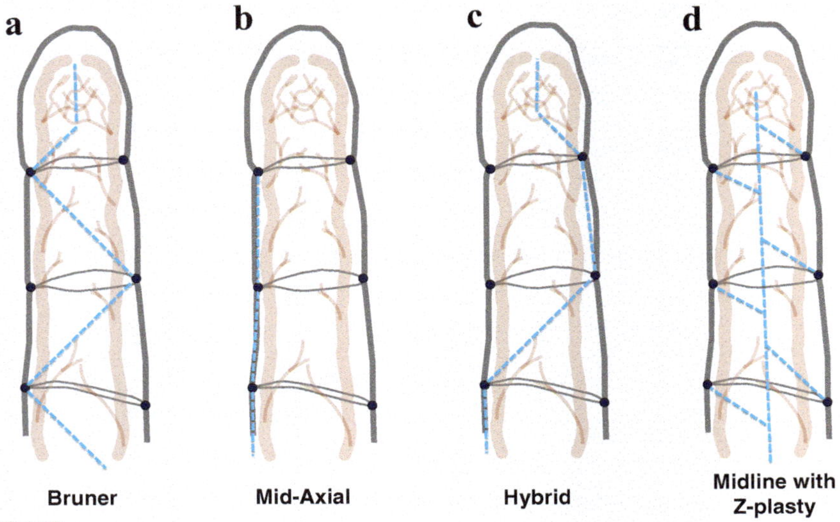

Fig. 14.1 Surgical incision options for Dupuytren's fasciectomy. Depending on cord morphology different incisions may offer a simpler dissection or broader exposure. If principles are obeyed, a variety of strategies can be used. (**a**) Bruner-style incision. (**b**) Mid-axial. (**c**) hybrid Bruner/mid-axial design. (**d**) Midline incision with z-plasty extensions

Table 14.1 Comparison of different volar digit approaches. It is difficult to say one approach is inherently better, but each technique has pros and cons in terms of exposure, surgical complexity, operative time, and long-term sequelae

	Midlateral Incision	Midline Incision with Z-Plasty	Bruner Incision
Exposure time	+	+	++
Closure time	+	+++	++
Ease of exposure for midline structures	+	+++	+++
Resultant scar location placement	Lateral digit	Volar digit	Volar digit
Impact on sensation	Dorsal branches of digital nerve potentially sacrificed	None	None
Risk of flap necrosis/flap tip necrosis	None	++	+

14.3 Skin Flap Physiology

Effective flap surgery requires thoughtfully placed incisions and dissection to allow for mobility of tissues while preserving sufficient blood supply to ensure viability [7]. For this reason, flap surgery is essentially the application of the micro- and macrovascular anatomy of a given region. Although flaps in Dupuytren's surgery are small and require more excursion than larger reconstructive surgeries, applying similar principles permits better exposure, less complications, and more flexibility in incision design.

The skin has a rich vascular supply that can be categorized into two patterns: zones supplied by direct perforators, and zones of secondary perfusion that receive flow indirectly from these perforators through a supra-fascial or subdermal vascular plexus [8]. Areas that are supplied directly are termed *angiosomes* and are the basis for pedicle flaps (i.e., radial forearm flaps). These territories are akin to dermatomes but form a more irregular patchwork over the body in comparison to the linear arrangement of neurologic domains.

Areas that receive perfusion secondarily are the basis of "random pattern flaps" which are described primary on the movement of the tissue (i.e., transposition, rotation, advancement) [7, 8]. Although there are many interconnections, blood flows primarily from a source artery through the subdermal vascular plexus [9]. This is the type of flap that is typically used in Dupuytren's incision design.

Principle 1
DUPUYTREN'S FLAPS ARE RANDOM PATTERN FLAPS AND SHOULD BE KEPT FULL THICKNESS TO CAPTURE THE SUBDERMAL VASCULAR PLEXUS.

As incisions are made and the subdermal plexus is disrupted, the proportion of blood flow from neighboring domains is reduced (Fig. 14.2). Fortunately, normal cutaneous perfusion exceeds metabolic needs due to the skin's role in thermoregulation [10], allowing portions of vascularity to be safely removed without jeopardizing viability [11]. Accepted limitations of flap geometry dictates that the length of a flap should not be greater than its width (i.e., 1:1 ratio) to ensure that perfusion pressures are able to supply the extent of the flap [7, 9, 11] (Fig. 14.3). This strict ratio is considered safe throughout the body, with areas of higher vascularity, such as the hand and face, being able to tolerate larger ratios, although risk of flap tip necrosis increases. [7]

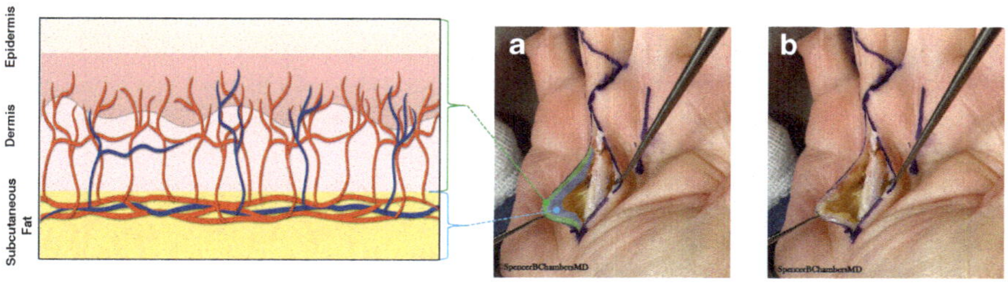

Fig. 14.2 Subdermal plexus location. When making incisions it is critical to protect the subdermal plexus which is the primary supply to flaps elevated in Dupuytren's surgery. This plexus is in the subcutaneous fat, making it critical to ensure that where possible skin flaps are elevated full thickness. (**a**) Pictorial diagram showing location of vascular plexus. (**b** and **c**) Clinical appearance of full-thickness skin flaps demonstrating the epidermis/dermis and subdermal fat containing the plexus

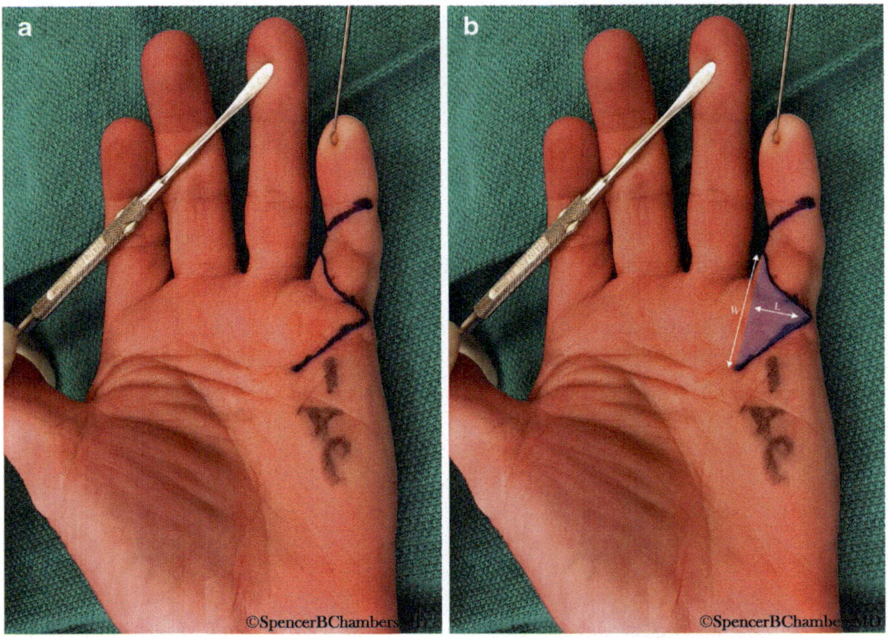

Fig. 14.3 Flap length and width design. When approaching single digits (**a**) as the intrinsic design of Bruner style flaps or Z-plasties intrinsically ensures the width of the base of the flap is greater than its length (**b**)

Principle 2
DESIGN FLAPS TO MAINTAIN A LENGTH-TO-WIDTH RATIO OF 1:1 TO ENSURE FLAP VIABILITY.

As redundant blood flow is removed, the tissue experiences transient ischemia, and maintenance of vascularity is reliant on the remaining source arteries [11]. This flow occurs through either true vascular connections, which are vessels of a fixed caliber, or through *choke anastomoses* [12]. A choke anastomoses is a capillary bed that normally has little blood flow but dilates in the setting of hypoxia. If the transient ischemia is not too great to completely compromise tissue viability, homeostatic pathways induce dilation of choke anastomoses to redirect flow through remaining channels while new vascular connections are produced [12]. This intermediate stage is critical with survival dependent on a low pressure and low flow state. Additional stressors such as external pressure or excess tension during wound closure should be avoided to optimize perfusion.

Principle 3
RANDOM PATTERN FLAPS ARE DEPENDENT ON PERFUSION PRESSURE FOR FLOW AND EXCESS EXTERNAL PRESSURE SHOULD BE AVOIDED.

Using these three principles, skin flaps are designed with broad bases to maximize inflow from remaining vessels, elevated in a uniform subcutaneous thickness to ensure the subdermal plexus is preserved, and closed with minimal tension to ensure remaining vascularity is not compressed (Fig. 14.4).

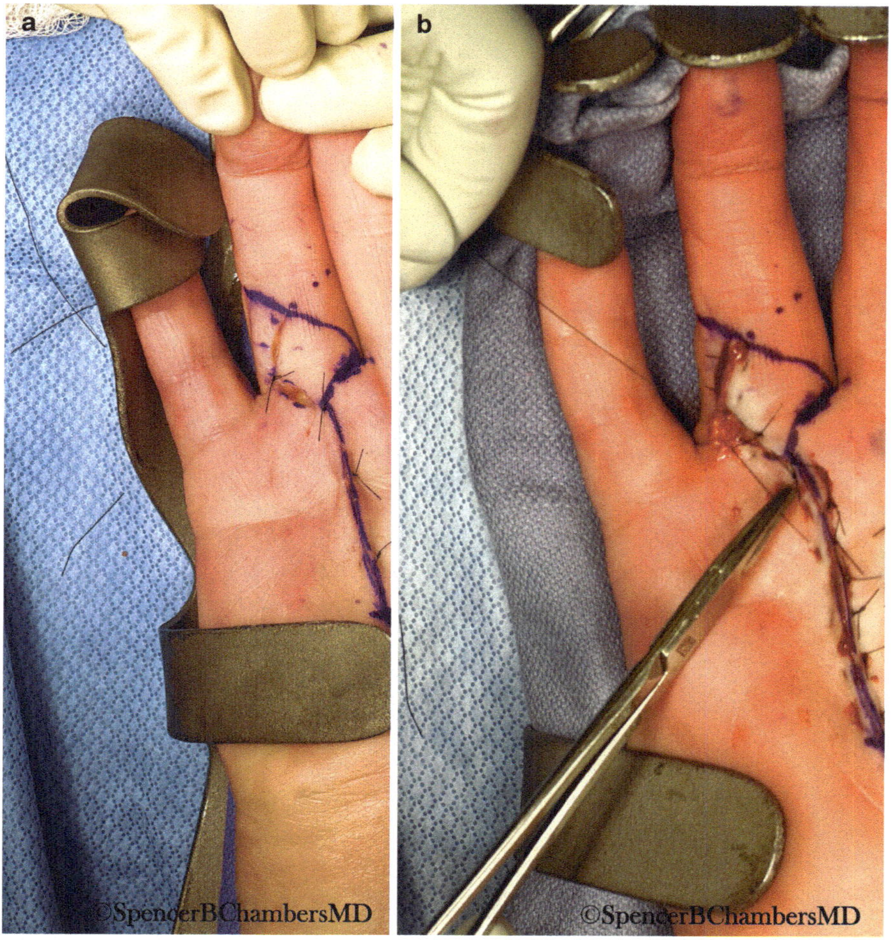

Fig. 14.4 Flap tip compression. When closing care must be taken not to apply too much tension or apply too much compression over flaps. Although horizontal mattresses are often preferential for closure to achieve dermal opposition, simple sutures at the tips of flaps, or judicious tightening should be considered. The above figure demonstrates a simple suture tensioned appropriately (**a**) compared to a horizontal mattress that is overtightened resulting in skin blanching and risking flap tip necrosis (**b**)

14.4 Wound Healing and Scar Formation

The normal stages of wound healing have been well described and include hemostasis, inflammation, proliferation, and remodeling [13]. Both hemostasis and inflammation are critical in the initial stages of injury to minimize blood loss and sterilize the wound. Proliferation follows with fibroblasts migrating to the wound to produce type 3 collagen to fill the defect [13]. After a preliminary collagen network has been produced, fibroblasts transform to myofibroblasts and wound contraction begins [14]. Given the abnormal fibroblast function in patients with Dupuytren's disease, in some cases this can also result in hypertrophic or thickened scars [15].

Wound healing is metabolically costly [16], making a reduction in wound size advantageous. However, this process can distort local tissues and when incisions cross areas of mobility, it leads to contracture (Fig. 14.5) [17, 18]. Even as the wound completes the final stages of remodeling and scar tissue becomes more supple, the shortened wound persists. Contracture is a particularly difficult problem in the fingers due to numerous joints and the large disability that small changes in range of motion can produce [18, 19].

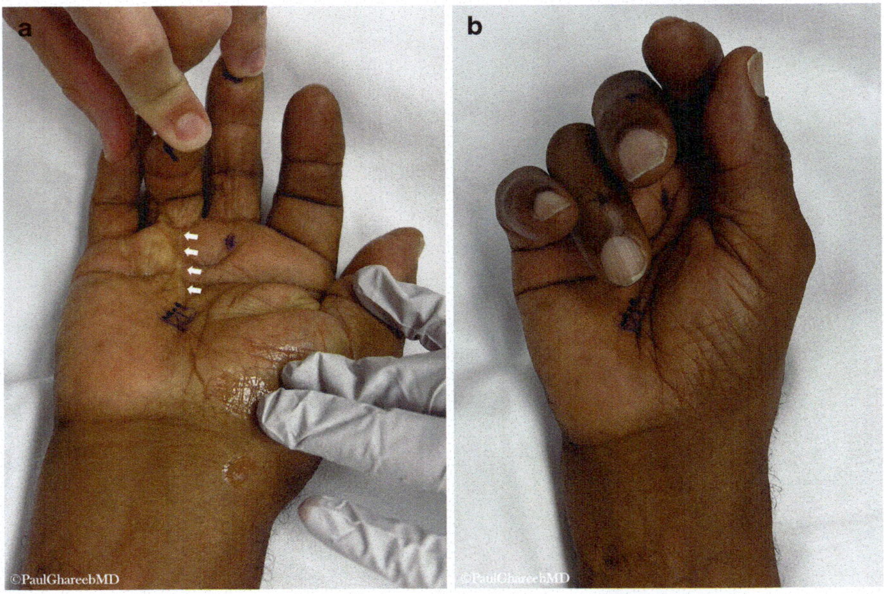

Fig. 14.5 Finger contracture secondary to longitudinal scar. As a normal healing process all scars will contract to make wounds smaller and less biologically costly to close. All wounds contract proportionally, with longer portions of an incision resulting in more shortening than short incisions. (**a**) demonstrates a longitudinal scar (white arrows) perpendicular to the axis of the metacarpophalangeal joint resulting in a contracture (**b**) and disturbance in cascade

Principle 4
WOUNDS CONTRACT DURING NORMAL HEALING POTENTIALLY PRODUCING CONTRACTURES IF INCISIONS CROSS REGIONS OF HIGH MOBILITY.

14.5 Principles of Skin Flap Design and Historical Perspective

The ideal surgical incision should maximize exposure, while minimizing disturbance to nerves, lymphatics, tendon gliding, and joint motion [1, 2].With critical neurovascular structures residing on the sides of each digit, the most simple and intuitive approach to accomplish this is a midline longitudinal incision [20, 21]. This was the case of early hand surgery that focused on management of infections, where incisions were positioned over a nidus to facilitate the most thorough debridement possible [21]. With significant risk of morbidity and mortality for inadequately treated infections, secondary complications from these incisions were a minor consideration [18]. As anesthesia and infection management improved, elective hand surgery flourished, necessitating a critical evaluation of the outcomes of these incisions, and the development of techniques that had more consideration for long-term function.Incisions crossing flexion creases in a perpendicular fashion were at high risk of contracture leading to disability [18]. These were areas of mobility described by Burton as diamond-shaped zones that should not be violated with longitudinal incisions (Fig. 14.6) [22].

Principle 5
BURTON'S DIAMONDS ARE THE AREAS OF HIGHEST MOBILITY IN THE DIGIT.

Conversely, incisions that were parallel to flexion creases posed the smallest risk of contracture, but greatest risk of iatrogenic injury to underlying structures. Balancing these conflicting tenants has produced 3 primary approaches to flap design historically:

14.5.1 Midlateral Incisions

Boyes first described mid-lateral incision to access the flexor tendon for treatment of pyogenic flexor tenosynovitis [20]. An incision was designed along the midlateral aspect of one side of the digit, joining isometric points over the interphalangeal

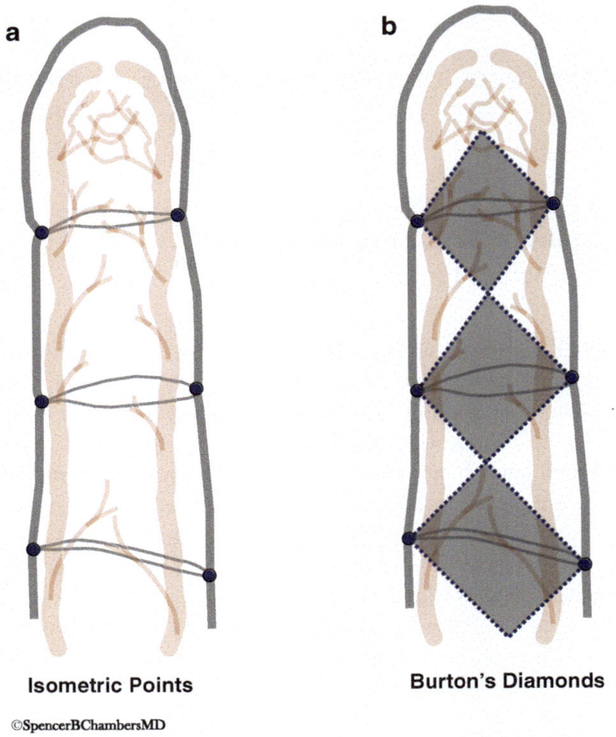

Fig. 14.6 Fixed points and areas of mobility in the digit. Isometric points represent areas that are stationary relative to one another throughout motion. Regardless of joint position, the distance will be fixed, implying that incisions connecting these points cannot be shortened. The converse is areas of mobility, which are defined as diamonds on the volar finger created by drawing lines joining these isometric points. (**a**) Isometric midlateral points. (**b**) Areas of skin mobility described by Burton

joints and dissecting dorsal to the neurovascular bundle. This produced a volar flap that was vascularized by the digital arteries, but elevation required transection of the dorsal branches of the digital nerves. This incision is expansile, and does not violate the volar skin, minimizing discomfort during postoperative rehabilitation and making contracture unlikely [23]. A modification to this incision was proposed by Koch and Mason where the incision was placed volar to the neurovascular structures (anterolateral) which produced easier access to volar structures but increased the risk of migration of the incision volarly potentially leading to secondary contracture [4].

14.5.2 Bruner Incisions

Julien Bruner advocated for a "zigzag" incision that has become popular in contemporary surgery and bears his name (Fig. 14.7) [1]. By connecting similar points to the mid-lateral incision but traversing the volar digit on the borders of Burton's diamonds, triangular flaps are created that can be elevated superficial to the

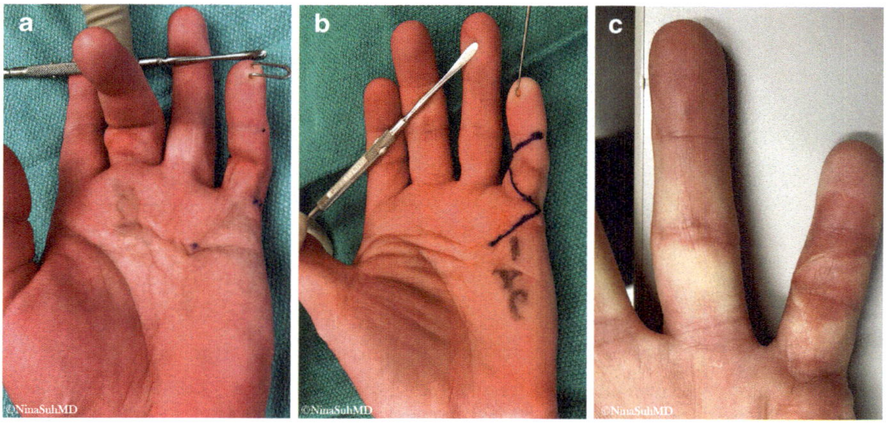

Fig. 14.7 Clinical application of isometric points. Beginning skin flap design by marking out the isometric points at the interphalangeal and metacarpophalangeal joints (**a**) is a simple approach to avoid incisions that may cause contracture (**b**). Bruner incisions are a workhorse flap design that allows broad exposure of underlying structures while producing flat cosmetic scars (**c**)

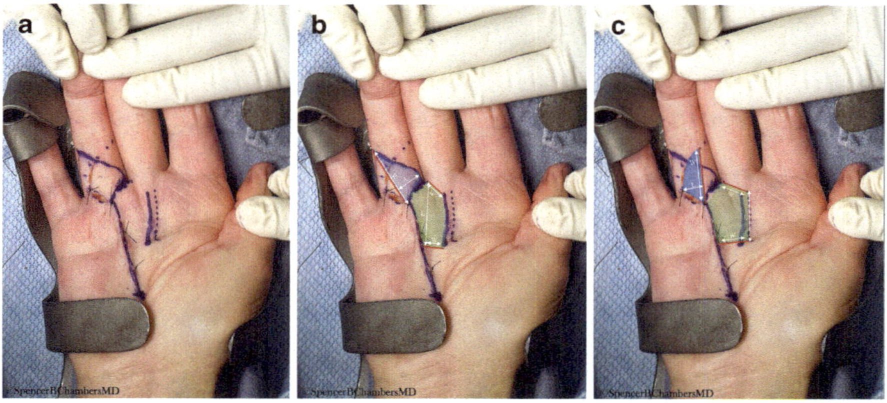

Fig. 14.8 Flap design optimization. When planning multiple digits or counter incisions, there are often at least two options with one being optimal. (**a**) Demonstrates two potential options (solid and dotted lines) for excision of disease in neighboring digits with option 1 (**b**) results in narrower based flaps compared to the latter option (**c**) which will produce more robust flaps

neurovascular and tendinous structures [22]. The flaps remain vascularized and innervated as long as the flaps are elevated full thickness. With no incisions crossing the flexure creases perpendicularly, secondary contracture is unlikely. Additionally, if required, a V-Y advancement can be carried out at the apex of each flap to increase scar length [6]. There is more planning required for extension than a midlateral incision, as there are two mirrored options possible for each digit. Other important considerations include ensuring that skin lesions that are planned for excision are positioned at the tip of the flap to ensure flap vascularity is not compromised by their removal, and coordinating incisions of multiple adjacent digits to maximize the width of the resultant webspace flaps (Fig. 14.8).

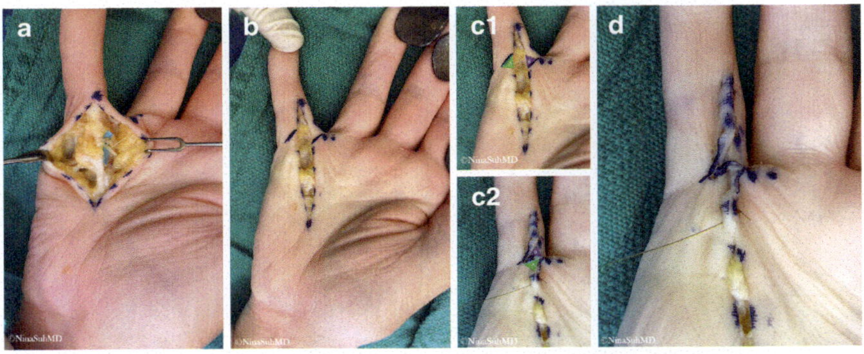

Fig. 14.9 Z-plasty scar manipulation after midline longitudinal incision. At times a midline incision facilitates a safe expansile approach (**a**). To avoid secondary contractures z-plasty advancement flaps can be created over each joint crossed (**b**). These flaps are transposed ($\mathbf{c}_1$ and $\mathbf{c}_2$) breaking up the straight midline scar (**d**)

Principle 6
IF A BRUNER INCISION DESIGN IS USED AND AN AREA OF SKIN IS PLANNED FOR EXCISION, THIS AREA SHOULD BE POSITIONED AT THE TIP OF THE FLAP.

14.5.3 Central Incisions with Z-Plasty

An alternative approach to preventing secondary contracture was attributed to McIndoe. Burton's diamonds were traversed with a midline incision to optimize visualization and speed, but later modified with z-plasty transposition flaps at each flexion crease at the completion of the excision to avoid secondary contracture (Fig. 14.9) [24]. A simple midline incision is easiest to perform in significant disease where an underlying contracture limits access to the distal digit. Exposure can be obtained proximally allowing a fasciotomy to improve mobility of the digit before progressing distally. Another variation to this technique is the elevation of Z-plasty flaps after developing a plane between the subcutaneous tissues and deeper structures prior to disease excision. This allows skin flaps to be retracted more fully for broader exposure but limits flexibility in placement of flaps.

14.6 Special Considerations in Skin Flap Design

14.6.1 Revision Surgery

In the setting of revision surgery, the safest exposure is to use the prior incision. Re-elevation ensures the most robust vascularity, although neovascularization in random pattern flaps from surrounding incisions and deep tissues has been demonstrated to occur as quickly as 7 days [9, 11]. If the original incision needs to be modified, keeping the base of new flaps broad and limiting deep dissection is advisable. Additionally, limiting vasospastic agents and observing flap color and cap refill during surgery is beneficial.

14.6.2 Patients with Early Arthritis and Skin Deficit

Elderly patients with concomitant arthritis and fascial disease are common. Postoperative stiffness is a major concern in this population and if adequate mobilization and splinting is not carried out postoperatively, results may be poor. For significant disease in the palm with an anticipated skin deficit (Fig. 14.10), an alternative approach can be used that was popularized by McCash [25]. A transverse incision in the palm is used to gain access to proximal disease which is excised. This incision is left open resulting in an elliptical wound that heals by secondary intention. There are no postoperative limitations on mobility and rehabilitation can begin immediately. If access to the digit is required additional transverse incisions in the interphalangeal flexion creases are used. These are closed primarily, and the larger wound in the palm heals after 6–8 weeks.

In other situations where disease has significant skin involvement requiring excision, skin grafting can be considered (Fig. 14.11), although this limits postoperative mobility and has a higher risk of postoperative hematoma [25].

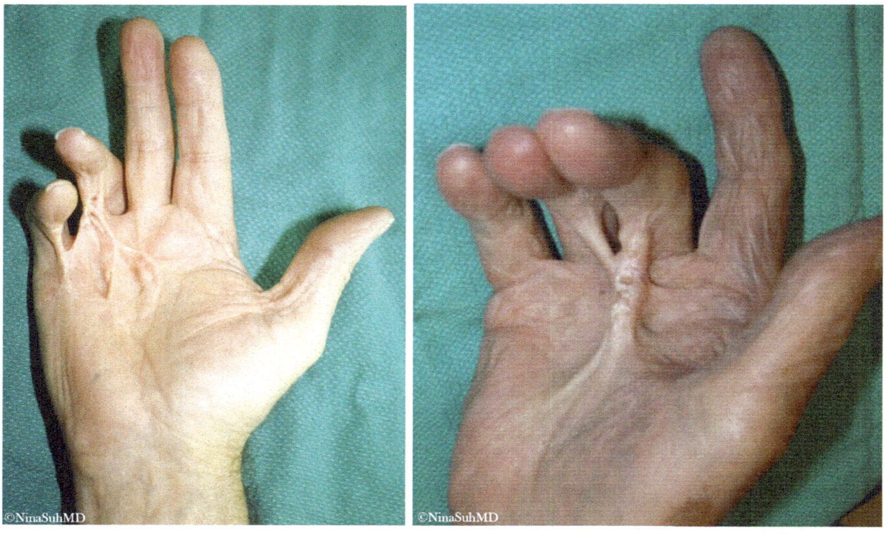

Fig. 14.10 Severe Dupuytren's disease with potential skin deficit. Even with thoughtful skin flap design, some significant diseases may have skin deficits requiring an open palm technique or secondary grafting in addition soft tissue flaps

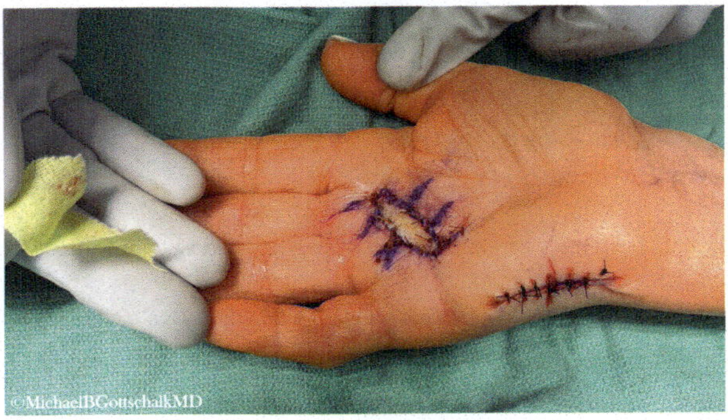

Fig. 14.11 Skin graft from hypothenar eminence. Pending the amount of skin deficit, the hypothenar eminence, volar wrist, or volar forearm often supply adequate coverage. Alternatively, open wounds can be managed conservatively, although time to closure may be increased

Table 14.2 Principles of flap elevation. Regardless of the surgical approach preferred, basic tenants derived from fundamental physiology, wound healing, and historical perspectives

Principles of flap design in the digit	
Principle 1	Dupytren's flaps are random pattern flaps and should be kept full thickness to capture the subdermal vascular
Principle 2	Design flaps to maintain a length-to-width ratio of 1:1 to ensure flap viability
Principle 3	Random pattern flaps are dependent on perfusion pressure for flow and excess external pressure should be avoided
Principle 4	Wounds contract during normal healing potentially producing contractures if incisions cross regions of high mobility
Principle 5	Burton's diamonds are the areas of highest mobility in the digit
Principle 6	If a Bruner incision design is used and an area of skin is planned for excision, this area should be positioned at the tip of the flap

14.6.3 Webspace Contracture

Dupuytren's disease impacting the webspace can cause limitations in gripping, particularly if the first webspace is involved. The underlying pathologic structure is the natatory chord [26]. The initial approach should involve a transverse incision over the webspace for excision of the deeper structures, and this incision can then be reoriented with serial z-plasties, double opposing z-plasties, or a jumping man flap [27]. The webspace can be splinted to further limit secondary shortening and contracture.

14.7 Conclusions

Incision design and flap elevation in Dupuytren's surgery is as diverse as the disease being treated. With an understanding of skin physiology, wound healing characteristics, and historic lessons of areas of tissue mobility, a variety of techniques can be successfully implemented (Table 14.2). Although a single technique is not intrinsically the best, if isometric points are joined in a manner that does not cross flexion perpendicularly and skin flaps are elevated to maintain vascularity, a surgeon has freedom to employ creativity in the incisions design during excision of this disease.

References

1. Bruner J. The zig-zag volar-digital incision for flexor-tendon surgery. Plast Reconstr Surg. 1967;40(6):571–4.
2. Bruner J. Incisions for plastic and reconstructive (non-septic) surgery of the hand. Br J Plast Surg. 1951;4(1):48–55.
3. Watson J. Fasciotomy and Z-plasty in the management of Dupuytren ' s contracture. Br J Plast Surg. 1984;37:27–30.
4. Hall RF, Vliegenthart DH. A modified midlateral incision for volar approach to the digit. J Hand Surg Am. 1986;11(2):195–7. https://doi.org/10.1016/0266-7681(86)90258-5.
5. Jobe MT, Caviale P, Milford LW. The digital palmar oblique incision. J Hand Surg Am. 1993;18(3):525–7. https://doi.org/10.1016/0363-5023(93)90106-D.
6. King EW, Exeter NH, Bass DM, Watson HK. Treatment of Dupuytren's contracture by extensive fasciectomy through multiple Y-V-plasty incisions: short-term evaluation of 170 consecutive operations. J Hand Surg Am. 1979;4(3):234–41. https://doi.org/10.1016/S0363-5023(79)80158-6.
7. Rehim SA, Chung K. Local flaps of the hand. Hand Clin. 2014;30(2):137–51. https://doi.org/10.1016/j.hcl.2013.12.004.Local.
8. Taylor G, Palmer J. The vascular territories (angiosomes) of the body: an experimental study and clinical implications. Br J Plast Surg. 1987;40:113.
9. Cormack G, Lamberty B. The arterial anatomy of skin flaps. 2nd ed. Churchill Livingstone; 1994.
10. Oberg P. Laser-doppler flowmetry. Crit Rev Biomed Eng. 1990;18(2):125–63.
11. Tsur H, Daniller A, Strauch B. Neovascularization of skin flaps: route and timing. Plast Reconstr Surg. 1980;66(1):85–94.
12. Toshiharu M, et al. The function of "choke vessels" to the blood flow: angiographic and laser flow-graphic study on the rat flap model. Int J Tissue Repair Regen. 2008;12(1):A15.
13. Gurtner GC, Werner S, Barrandon Y, Longaker MT. Wound repair and regeneration. Nature. 2008;453(7193):314–21. https://doi.org/10.1038/nature07039.
14. Desmoulière A, Chaponnier C, Gabbiani G. Tissue repair, contraction, and the myofibroblast. Wound Repair Regen. 2005;13(1):7–12. https://doi.org/10.1111/j.1067-1927.2005.130102.x.
15. Rivlin M, Osterman M, Jacoby SM, Skirven T, Ukomadu U, Osterman AL. The incidence of postoperative flare reaction and tissue complications in Dupuytren's disease using tension-free immobilization. Hand. 2014;9(4):459–65. https://doi.org/10.1007/s11552-014-9638-6.
16. Long CL, Schaffel N, Geiger JW, Schiller WR, Blakemore WS. Metabolic response to injury and illness: estimation of energy and protein needs from indirect calorimetry and nitrogen balance. J Parenter Enter Nutr. 1979;3(6):452–6. https://doi.org/10.1177/014860717900300609.
17. Davis JS, Kitlowski EA. The theory and prafticał use of the Z-incision for the relief of scar contractures. Ann Surg. 1939;109(6):1001–15. https://doi.org/10.1201/b17524-6.
18. Bunnell S. Contractures of the hand from infections and injuries. J Bone Jt Surg. 1932;14:27–46.
19. Moran SL, Berger RA. Biomechanics and hand trauma: what you need. Hand Clin. 2003;19(1):17–31. https://doi.org/10.1016/S0749-0712(02)00130-0.
20. Boyes J. Incisions in the hand. Am J Orthop. 1962;4:308–11.
21. Kanavel A, Mason M. Infections of the hand. FA Davis; 1939.
22. Burton S. Principals of surgery. 4th ed. McGraw-Hill; 1984.

23. Dancey A, Titley OG. A modification of the Bruner incision for the hand and review of the literature. J Plast Reconstr Aesthetic Surg. 2008;61(9):1130–1. https://doi.org/10.1016/j.bjps.2008.05.004.
24. Bruner JM. The contributions of Sir Archibald McIndoe to surgery of the hand. Ann R Coll Surg Engl. 1973;53(1):1–12.
25. McCash C. The open palm techniquer in Dupytrens contracture. Br J Plast Surg. 1964;17:271.
26. Milner RH. Dupuytren's disease affecting the thumb and first web of the hand. J Hand Surg Am. 2003;28 B(1):33–6. https://doi.org/10.1054/jhsb.2002.0840.
27. McGregor I. The Z- plasty in han surgery. J Bone Jt Surg. 1967;49(B):448–57.

Chapter 15
Skin Grafting: How and When to Do It

Christine V. Schaeffer

15.1 Introduction

Dupuytren's disease is a progressive disease without a curative treatment to date. The procedures described for management of finger flexion contractures range from the limited release of Dupuytren's cords to radical dermofasciectomy with or without skin graft. The presence of myofibroblasts within the palmar aponeurosis is thought to contribute to clinical Dupuytren's contractures [1]. Histologic studies have identified myofibroblasts within the overlying dermis and subcutaneous tissue in patients with Dupuytren's disease, which may contribute to recurrent disease following limited fasciectomies [2, 3]. These studies suggested a potential benefit to skin excision in the management of severe or recurrent Dupuytren's disease. Dermofasciectomy was first described by Hueston in 1962 as a technique to reduce recurrence rates of Dupuytren's disease. This approach involves excision of the Dupuytren's cords in addition to the overlying skin followed by application of a full-thickness skin graft (FTSG) [4]. This chapter will describe the indications, considerations, surgical technique, and the risks/outcomes of dermofasciectomy with FTSG.

15.2 Indications

The classically described applications for full-thickness grafts in the setting of Dupuytren's disease include large grafts for dermofasciectomy defects (Fig. 15.1), small grafts used as "firebreaks" (Fig. 15.2), and grafts for skin deficits following limited fasciectomy [4–6]. Dermofasciectomy with FTSG is primarily indicated in

C. V. Schaeffer (✉)
University of Kentucky Plastic & Reconstructive Surgery, Lexington, KY, USA

M. B. Gottschalk et al. (eds.), *Dupuytren's Disease*,
https://doi.org/10.1007/978-3-031-85873-4_15

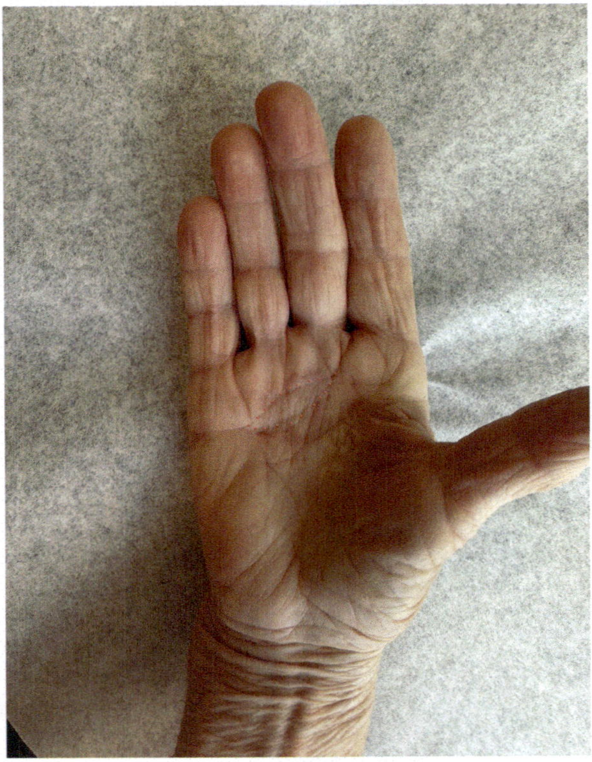

Fig. 15.1 Dermofasciectomy with application of full-thickness skin graft for recurrent Dupuytren's disease with extensive skin involvement (outlined in red)

patients with high risk of recurrence and in the setting of recurrent disease with diffuse skin involvement. However, it has also been described as a primary procedure for select patients with marked Dupuytren's diathesis [7, 8]. Additional indications for FTSG include dermofasciectomy with the skin defect overlying the proximal phalanx and in the setting of severe proximal interphalangeal joint flexion contractures [9–11].

15.3 Considerations for Management of Recurrent Dupuytren's Disease

Historically, the leading indication for dermofasciectomy with FTSG was in the setting of recurrent Dupuytren's disease with extensive skin involvement [7]. Recurrent disease with well-defined cords may be amenable to percutaneous needle aponeurotomy or collagenase injection [9]. Vlot reports rates of contracture correction and recurrence to be similar between primary and secondary percutaneous needle aponeurotomies and third and fourth treatments [12]. Open treatment options include

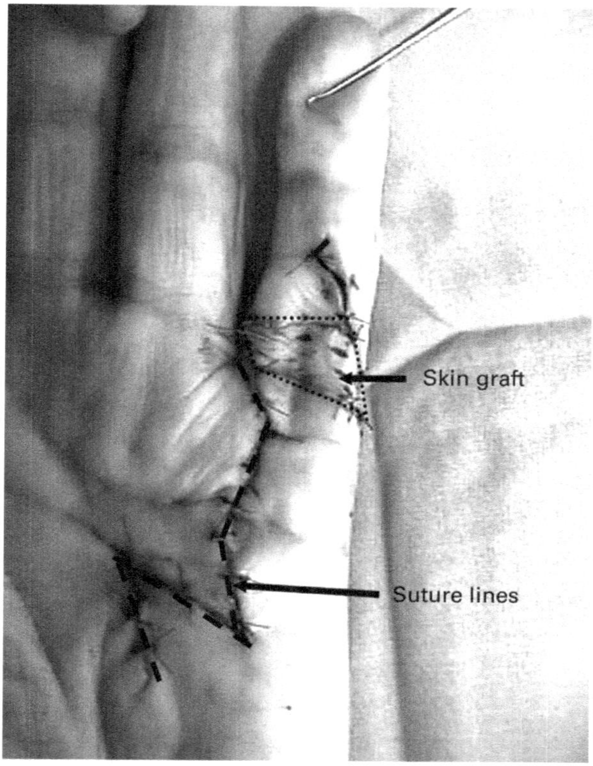

Fig. 15.2 "Firebreak" Graft demonstrated by Ullah et al. Small area of skin is excised with application of fenestrated full-thickness skin graft over the resulting skin defect. Note amount of skin excision is significantly less than classically described radical dermofasciectomy

limited fasciectomy, dermofasciectomy with FTSG, and an open palm technique (e.g., McCash). The potential benefits of these open approaches in recurrent disease include improved visualization of the altered anatomy from prior surgery and associated scar burden [13]. An open approach is preferred in the setting of more poorly defined Dupuytren's disease causing the recurrent contracture and in the setting of severe joint contractures that will likely require periarticular release [9]. A recently published meta-analysis demonstrated a lack of consensus regarding the most effective treatment for recurrent Dupuytren's disease [14].

In a recent systematic review of the literature, dermatofasciectomy with FTSG was the most commonly performed procedure as a revision operation (followed by open palm technique) [7]. A retrospective review of revision procedures for recurrent Dupuytren's disease in 33 patients at a single institution reported that 72% underwent partial fasciectomy, while 23% underwent dermofasciectomy. Additionally, 43% of patients required full-thickness skin grafts. The average size of the skin grafts required was 7.1 cm^2 [10].

15.4 Proposed Benefits of FTSG

The use of a full thickness skin graft in the setting of skin deficiency facilitates tension-free wound closure, thereby downregulating the activity of myofibroblasts and decreasing rates of recurrence [15]. Previous studies in animal models have demonstrated that full-thickness skin grafts accelerate ("burn out") myofibroblast lifecycles within the wound bed [16, 17]. Small full-thickness grafts, referred to as "firebreak" grafts, have been described to be placed over flexion creases (Fig. 15.2). This term alludes to the graft's ability to prevent disease recurrence by bringing in skin from a location free of Dupuytren's disease [5, 18].

Recurrence rates following procedures for management Dupuytren's disease vary significantly in the literature due to inconsistent definitions of a "recurrence" and variable lengths of follow-up [14]. Based on the previously cited histologic studies, excision of the skin overlying the Dupuytren's cords may decrease the risk of recurrence. The current literature regarding the influence of FTSG on Dupuytren's recurrence rates remains mixed.

15.4.1 Recurrence After Dermofasciectomy with FTSG

Ketchum and Hixson reported no recurrent disease beneath the graft in 36 hands following dermofasciectomy and application of FTSG with 8% of patients having disease progression of disease outside of the grafted area at an average of 3.9 years of follow-up [19]. In a retrospective review of 18 patients with bilateral, recurrent Dupuytren's disease, dermofasciectomy with FTSG was performed on 23 rays. In the hands that underwent FTSG, only 3 recurrences were noted at 8 years follow-up (13%); recurrence occurred in all instances (27 rays) where FTSG was not performed [20]. In a recent systematic review of the literature including 79 studies, recurrence rate was the lowest following dermofasciectomy with FTSG (6.3% with dermofasciectomy with FTSG, 19% with limited fasciectomy, and 20.3% with open palm technique). Of note, the average follow-up was 4.9 years, 4.1 years, and 4.0 years, respectively. The majority of studies included in this review were case series with a high risk of bias [7].

15.4.2 Recurrence After Dermofasciectomy with Firebreak FTSG Graft

A randomized control study in 2009 was performed to evaluate recurrence rate following dermofasciectomy with firebreak FTSG vs limited fasciectomy in patients with primary Dupuytren's contractures. There was no difference in recurrence rates at 3 years between the two groups (13.6% vs 10.9%, respectively; $p = 0.7$) [21]. In a retrospective review of 47 patients who underwent dermofasciectomy with FTSG, the indication for surgery was recurrent disease in 35 patients and primary contracture in 12 patients. There were no cases of recurrent disease beneath the graft at an average of 8.4 years of follow-up, however there was evidence of disease progression outside of the operative area in 83% of cases. Interestingly, all 12 patients who underwent dermofasciectomy and FTSG for primary contracture had disease progression. In this study, the risk of progression of Dupuytren's disease outside of the operative area following dermofasciectomy and FTSG was noted to be associated with severity of Dupuytren's disease [22].

In addition to recurrent disease, cases have been reported of Dupuytren's disease status post dermofasciectomy and FTSG with recurrent flexion contracture in addition to infiltration of the full thickness skin grafts by Dupuytren's disease on histologic evaluation [23].

15.5 Detriments of FTSG

There is a wide range of procedures described for the management of primary and recurrent Dupuytren's contractures. When compared to less invasive techniques (i.e., percutaneous needle aponeurotomy and collagenase injection), procedures that involve full-thickness skin grafting are more invasive and therefore have higher risk of nerve injury, longer post-operative recovery, and increased scar burden [9]. The largest dissection, resection, and skin graft are required following dermofasciectomy when compared to limited fasciectomy and fasciectomy with skin grafts [13].

15.6 Outcomes/Complications

A systematic review of the literature on outcomes for surgical interventions in European patients (48 articles) demonstrated high rates of nerve injuries, infection, and hematomas associated with dermofasciectomy with FTSG compared to limited fasciectomy [24]. In the randomized control study by Ullah et al., there was no significant difference in post-operative complications between patients who underwent limited fasciectomy vs dermofasciectomy with firebreak graft [21]. Graft failure rates range in the literature from <1 to 8.6% [8, 11, 20, 25]. Ansari et al. report a mean post-operative satisfaction rate score of 7.7 out of 10 when dermofasciectomy with FTSG was performed as a primary procedure [11].

15.7 Technique and Post-operative Management

A template of the recipient site skin defect is used to guide the design of the skin graft. FTSG harvest is performed with a 15-blade scalpel from the ipsilateral antecubital fossa, ulnar forearm, or hypothenar eminence with primary closure of the donor site. Of note, the hypothenar eminence provides glabrous skin, and one can harvest up to 2 cm in width by 5 cm in length with primary closure of the donor site [13].

Arm tourniquets should be deflated at the time of graft inset to mitigate risk of hematoma formation and subsequent graft failure [26]. The graft is defatted and fenestrated to allow for fluid egress (Fig. 15.2). It is then secured with absorbable sutures to the recipient site and a bolster dressing is applied. The first dressing change (with bolster removal) is typically performed at 5–7 days post-surgery. The use of a non-adherent Mepitel dressing (Mölnlycke Health Care, Peachtree Corners, GA, USA) followed by gauze over the skin graft site has been described in lieu of bolster dressing [11, 27]. Another described alternative to bolstering of the skin graft is the use of quilting sutures along the midline of the graft into the underlying flexor tendon sheath following peripheral graft inset [28]. It is important to confirm unimpeded flexor tendon excursion following placement of these sutures. A recent study found that first dressing change at 48 hours followed by early range of motion was safe and did not significantly increase graft failure rates [11].

15.8 Conclusion

Dermatofasciectomy with full-thickness skin graft can be considered in recurrent Dupuytren's disease, especially in patients with extensive skin involvement. While FTSG does not prevent disease progression outside of the previous operative area, the rate of disease recurrence involving the graft is low compared to other described techniques (limited fasciectomy alone, open palm technique).

Grafts harvested outside of the palm have the theoretical benefit of bringing in tissue without the propensity to develop Dupuytren's disease. The author's preferred donor site is the medial forearm—this site is within the operative field, is relatively hairless, and can typically be closed primarily. A template of the defect is created using the foil of the suture packet for Chromic Gut suture (which will be used to inset the graft). This template is transposed to the graft donor site and full-thickness harvest is performed. It is key to de-fat the graft and fenestrate to allow for fluid egress. The author performs a tie-over bolster dressing with xeroform wrapped cotton balls with mineral oil that is removed on POD 5–7. Daily dressing changes with non-stick gauze and finger range of motion are then initiated.

References

1. Gabbiani G, Majno G. Dupuytren's contracture: fibroblast contraction? An ultrastructural study. Am J Pathol. 1972;66(1):131–46.
2. McCann BG, Logan A, Belcher H, Warn A, Warn RM. The presence of myofibroblasts in the dermis of patients with Dupuytren's contracture. A possible source for recurrence. J Hand Surg Br. 1993;18(5):656–61.
3. Chen W, Zhou H, Pan ZJ, Chen JS, Wang L. The role of skin and subcutaneous tissues in Dupuytren's contracture: an electron microscopic observation. Orthop Surg. 2009;1(3):216–21.
4. Hueston JT. Digital Wolfe grafts in recurrent Dupuytren's contracture. Plast Reconstr Surg Transplant Bull. 1962;29:342–4.
5. Hueston JT. Firebreak' grafts in Dupuytren's contracture. Aust N Z J Surg. 1984;54(3):277–81.
6. Crockett JE. Adequate fasciectomy and the use of full-thickness skin gussets in the treatment of Dupuytren's contracture. Ann R Coll Surg Engl. 1980;62(3):230–1.
7. De Ketele A, Degreef I. Full-thickness skin grafting in preventing recurrence of Dupuytren's disease: a systematic review. Hand Surg Rehabil. 2023;42(4):273–83.
8. Tonkin MA, Burke FD, Varian JP. Dupuytren's contracture: a comparative study of fasciectomy and dermofasciectomy in one hundred patients. J Hand Surg Br. 1984;9(2):156–62.
9. Kaplan FTD, Crosby NE. Treatment of recurrent Dupuytren disease. Hand Clin. 2018;34(3):403–15.
10. Hozack BA, Rayan GM. Surgical treatment for recurrent Dupuytren disease. Hand. 2023;18(4):641–7.
11. Ansari SA, Kennedy JA, Younis F. Skin graft review in dermofasciectomy for Dupuytren's contracture within 48 hours: challenging historical practice. J Hand Microsurg. 2022;14(1):71–8.
12. Vlot MAWP. Effectiveness of percutaneous needle fasciotomy for second or higher recurrence in Dupuytren contracture. Cham: Springer; 2017.
13. Draeger RW, Stern PJ. Recurrent Dupuytren contracture treated with fasciectomy and skin grafting. In: Rizzo M, editor. Dupuytren's contracture: a clinical casebook. Cham: Springer International Publishing; 2016. p. 253–66.
14. Wong CR, Huynh MNQ, Fageeh R, McRae MC. Outcomes of management of recurrent Dupuytren contracture: a systematic review and meta-analysis. Hand. 2022;17(6):1104–13.
15. Citron N, Hearnden A. Skin tension in the aetiology of Dupuytren's disease; a prospective trial. J Hand Surg Br. 2003;28(6):528–30.
16. Rudolph R, Suzuki M, Guber S, Woodward M. Control of contractile fibroblasts by skin grafts. Surg Forum. 1977;28:524–5.
17. Rudolph R. Inhibition of myofibroblasts by skin grafts. Plast Reconstr Surg. 1979;63(4):473–80.
18. Hueston JT. Dermofasciectomy for Dupuytren's disease. Bull Hosp Joint Dis Orthop Inst. 1984;44(2):224–32.
19. Ketchum LD, Hixson FP. Dermofasciectomy and full-thickness grafts in the treatment of Dupuytren's contracture. J Hand Surg Am. 1987;12(5 Pt 1):659–64.
20. Villani F, Choughri H, Pelissier P. Importance of skin graft in preventing recurrence of Dupuytren's contracture. Chir Main. 2009;28(6):349–51.
21. Ullah AS, Dias JJ, Bhowal B. Does a 'firebreak' full-thickness skin graft prevent recurrence after surgery for Dupuytren's contracture?: a prospective, randomised trial. J Bone Joint Surg Br. 2009;91(3):374–8.
22. Torrekens M, Van Nuffel M, Couck I, De Smet L, Degreef I. Skin grafting prevents recurrence in Dupuytren's disease and extension correlates with fibrosis diathesis score. Hand Surg Rehabil. 2021;40(4):495–9.
23. Wade RG, Igali L, Figus A. Dupuytren disease infiltrating a full-thickness skin graft. J Hand Surg Am. 2016;41(8):e235–8.
24. Crean SM, Gerber RA, Le Graverand MP, Boyd DM, Cappelleri JC. The efficacy and safety of fasciectomy and fasciotomy for Dupuytren's contracture in European patients: a structured review of published studies. J Hand Surg Eur. 2011;36(5):396–407.

25. Hall PN, Fitzgerald A, Sterne GD, Logan AM. Skin replacement in Dupuytren's disease. J Hand Surg Br. 1997;22(2):193–7.
26. Putnam J. Advanced Dupuytren contracture: approach to management. Hand Clin. 2023;39(3):455–63.
27. Tanagho A, Beaumont J, Thomas R. A simple dressing technique following dermofasciectomy and full thickness skin grafting of the fingers in the treatment of severe Dupuytren's contracture. J Hand Microsurg. 2015;7(2):317–9.
28. Akhavani MA, McKinnell T, Kang NV. Quilting of full thickness grafts in the hand. J Plast Reconstr Aesthet Surg. 2010;63(9):1534–7.

Chapter 16
Use of WALANT for Dupuytren's Contracture

Nathan Khabyeh-Hasbani and Steven M. Koehler

16.1 Introduction

The occurrence of Dupuytren's disease has been documented to reach up to 25% among males of Anglo-Saxon descent, with its likelihood rising as individuals age [1]. A majority of patients often opt to undergo surgery for the condition with Burke et al. reporting an occurrence rate of 32.5/100,000 years with 20.5/100,000 years opting for surgical fasciectomy [2].

Historically, procedures involving digital and palmar fasciectomy for Dupuytren's disease were commonly performed in the primary operating room with the patient under general anesthesia and using a tourniquet. In the past, the utilization of local anesthesia for this surgery was challenging due to two main limitations. The first was due to the requirement for an arm or forearm tourniquet, which awake patients found uncomfortable and painful when used for extended durations. The second was based off the dogma that, for nearly a century, it was widely taught that the use of epinephrine was not recommended for the "fingers, nose, penis, and toes" [3]. This theory was extrapolated from studies conducted in the early twentieth century, which demonstrated that a combination of procaine and epinephrine led to digital necrosis [4–7]. However, De Rougemont and Carcassoone documented 1500 cases of digital blocks involving epinephrine without any resulting digital necrosis and even observed instances of digital necrosis even in the absence of epinephrine use in digital blocks [8]. Following De Rougemont and Carcassonne's article, numerous subsequent studies also confirmed the safe utilization of epinephrine in local anesthetics, demonstrating that it could be employed without the occurrence of digital necrosis [9, 10]. One of the most renowned investigations that refuted this old dogma was the Dalhousie project by Lalonde et al.

N. Khabyeh-Hasbani · S. M. Koehler (✉)
Department of Orthopaedic Surgery, Montefiore Medical Center, Bronx, NY, USA
e-mail: nhasbani@montefiore.org; stkoehler@montefiore.org

M. B. Gottschalk et al. (eds.), *Dupuytren's Disease*,
https://doi.org/10.1007/978-3-031-85873-4_16

[11] which included a continuous series of 3110 cases involving epinephrine injection into the hands and fingers without the application of an arm tourniquet. This multicenter study provided evidence that during the period spanning from 2002 to 2004, a total of 203 consecutive Dupuytren's fasciectomies were carried out without the utilization of an arm tourniquet or general anesthesia and with no occurrences of ischemic complications [11]. Since Dr. Donald H. Lalonde first described the case of wide-awake local anesthesia with no tourniquet (WALANT) technique over a decade ago [12] there has been a shift in treating hand cases in the outpatient setting.

Since its introduction, WALANT has gained widespread recognition for its applicability across a growing range of hand and wrist procedures [13]. The promising clinical outcomes observed in routine surgeries like flexor tendon repair, tendon transfer, carpal tunnel release, and trigger finger release, contributed to the early popularity of WALANT [14–16]. Since then, the scope of procedures adopting this technique has expanded considerably to include arthroscopic and open wrist arthroscopy for triangular fibrocartilage repair [17], trapeziometacarpal joint prosthesis implantation [18], and even flap harvesting transfer in the hand [19].

In a retrospective analysis of 148 fingers subjected to treatment for Dupuytren's contracture, with 102 undergoing local anesthesia and 46 receiving general anesthesia, findings revealed no significant difference in terms of postoperative total active motion, changes in extension and complication rates between the two groups [20]. Nevertheless, the authors proposed that performing Dupuytren's fasciectomy using the wide-awake technique presents with a greater challenge due to the bleeding generated from adjacent cord dissection and as a result, preferred correction of Dupuytren's contracture under general anesthesia with the application of a tourniquet [20].

The objective of this chapter is to describe our successful surgical approach and strategies for addressing Dupuytren's contracture using the WALANT method.

16.2 Procedural Techniques and Methods

16.2.1 Procedural Description

On the day of the procedure, the surgeon can efficiently schedule multiple patients undergoing WALANT procedures due to minimal room cleanup following each procedure. In one study, the authors reported their team could complete nine carpal tunnel release procedures in a 3-hour period in the ambulatory setting compared to four in the main OR during the same time period [21]. When performing cases under WALANT, the surgical team typically consists of the surgeon, one assistant, and one circulating nurse. Our experience showed that the use of a single nurse, alongside the surgeon and assistant, in WALANT cases, yielded positive results contrary to common recommendations in many institutions which mandates the presence of two nurses during local anesthesia procedures [22]. By having a single nurse on the team, institutions have the potential to enhance nursing staffing across the facility, increase turnover efficiency, and lower costs per case.

Once patients have been welcomed by the administrative team, they proceed to our procedural suite for a consultation with the surgical team. The application of WALANT eliminates the necessity for anesthesia providers to be involved in securing surgical clearance, administering sedation, or overseeing patient monitoring [21, 23]. For procedures performed under WALANT, patients are exempted from such monitoring, with fasting prior to the procedure is no longer necessary, and halting of medications is not warranted [24, 25]. It is important to note that we do not stop anticoagulation.

Preoperatively, our approach involves performing peri-incisional injections along the marked incisional area to provide the hemostatic benefits of epinephrine. Our distinctive technique centers on the timing after the injection of local anesthesia and the initial incision.

In Dupuytren's surgery, there is always a concern for possible postoperative ischemia following correction due to vasospasm of the digital vessels. This exists irrespective of WALANT technique; however, it is certainly an accentuated concern of many surgeons due to the presence of epinephrine. This can be mitigated by careful injection technique and adherence to WALANT flap dissection principles [26]. There is extensive precedent for injecting epinephrine around microvascular structures. Wong et al. first described WALANT replantation in 12 cases in 2017 [27] by injecting at the level of the distal palmar crease and avoiding bathing the digital vessels in high volume of epinephrine. This permitted collateral flow. There is a fallacy that has been perpetuated that epinephrine affects the capillaries and not the larger vessels [19]. This is incorrect, as epinephrine has been shown to constrict the arterioles and the venules. The venular constriction is active and not secondary to the arteriolar constriction. There is no active capillary constriction with the use of epinephrine [28]. By keeping epinephrine away from flap pedicles, multiple authors have been successful in performing WALANT flaps [19, 26, 29]. Therefore, we advocate in our technique to also always perform injections in the palm, never in the fingers, and while peri-incisionally, avoid "bathing" the digital vessels in high volumes of epinephrine.

Following injection of the anesthetic, patients are instructed to spend a minimum of 45 min in our waiting room, which contrasts with the previously held belief that ~25 min suffices. While studies have indicated that ~25 min post-anesthetic injection is satisfactory for various hand procedures like carpal tunnel release [30], our WALANT protocol entails waiting 45–60 min following injection. This extended wait duration is essential to achieve a dry bloodless surgical field conducive to the meticulous dissection of the neurovascular bundle and the removal of Dupuytren's cords (Fig. 16.1). During this time, while one patient awaits the onset of anesthetic effects, the surgeon may also provide consultation to another patient undergoing WALANT and perform other procedures.

Our preference is to design Skoog-type incisions and then perform Z-plasties at the end of the procedure (Fig. 16.2a, b). This type of incisional pattern gives room to adjust the skin flaps. We place our Z-plasties between skin creases to prevent

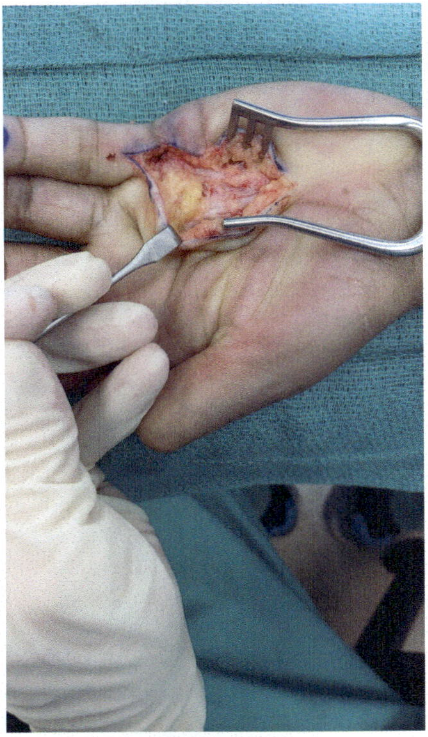

Fig. 16.1 Intraoperative visualization of the hemostatic effect of the epinephrine injection following our 45-min wait protocol

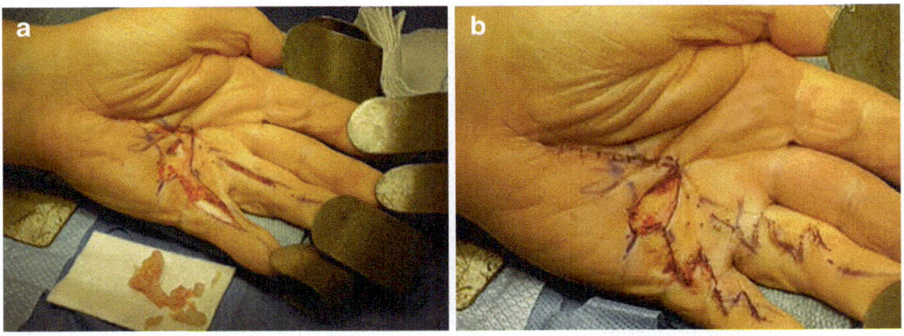

Fig. 16.2 (**a**) Skoog-type of incisions. (**b**): Z-plasty incisions

increased tension and decrease the risk of tip necrosis as there is much more laxity in these areas. In cases where there is skin shortage in the palm, we employ a McCash open palm technique, and the wound is left to heal by secondary intention. Postoperative splinting is very important in this technique to prevent contracture and patients are provided with "pancake" postoperative splints.

When performing WALANT dissections, we first make our incisions proximally and identify the neurovascular bundles (Fig. 16.3a, b). We then utilize tenotomy

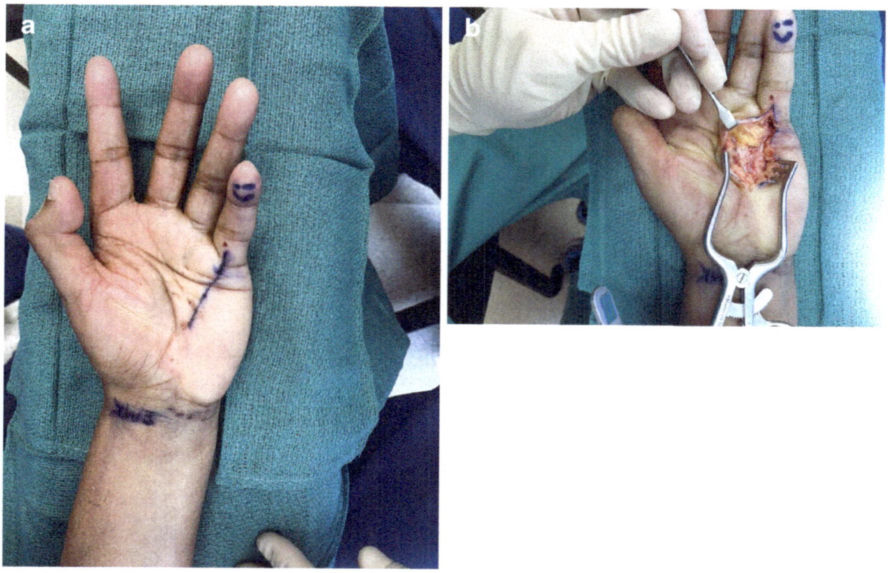

Fig. 16.3 (**a**): Patient undergoing left little finger correction of Dupuytren's contracture under WALANT. (**b**): Following incision and retraction, identification of the neurovascular bundle is visible

scissors which can be passed along the bundles, creating tunnels (Fig. 16.4). The walls of the tunnels are the septa of Legueu and Juvara, which are rarely involved in contractures and separate the neurovascular bundles from the flexor tendons. The cord lies over the flexor tendons and creates a "three-legged stool" between the two neurovascular bundles. By creating tunnels on the radial and ulnar neurovascular bundles and freeing the cord away from the bundles, the cord translates more midline and elevates volarly away from the flexor tendon, making it easier to dissect proximal to distal, visualizing the nerves more easily.

Intraoperative benefits of WALANT include evaluation of the strength and function of repairs and reductions through active patient participation, which has been associated with improved clinical outcomes [14, 31]. In Dupuytren's contractures, we employ WALANT to educate patients regarding postoperative wound care, splinting, and home exercise protocols. This is especially vital when the McCash technique is employed, and we rely on the patient for successful secondary intention.

Patients undergoing the wide-awake approach with pure local anesthesia do not suffer any postoperative nausea and vomiting, which on the contrary is usually estimated to occur in 20–40% of patients undergoing general anesthesia [32, 33]. Therefore, patients undergoing WALANT for correction of Dupuytren's contracture avoid the post-anesthesia care unit, leading to reduced hospitalization, prevention of admissions due to issues related to general anesthesia, and a quicker discharge for patients.

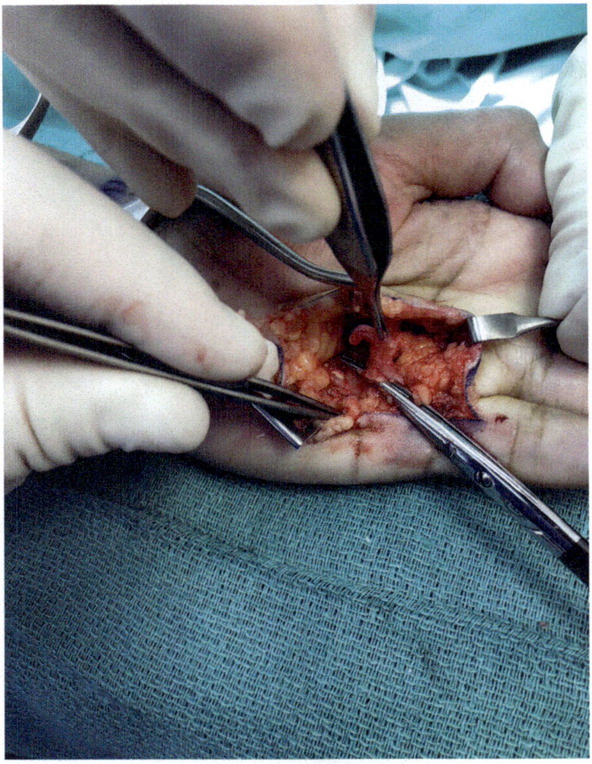

Fig. 16.4 Intraoperative depiction of tenotomy scissors passing along the bundles, creating tunnels

16.2.2 Field Prep Sterility

Since the procedure can be performed in an office setting, concerns might arise regarding the potential increased risk of infection due to the confined scope of sterility and draping. When performing WALANT procedures at our institution, meticulous field preparation for sterility is employed to minimize waste with limited instrumentation and maximal efficiency. For field sterility in the office, a single drape or four surgical towels, gloves, masks, and a sterile tray with limited instruments are needed (Fig. 16.5a, b). The use of gowns, excessive draping, and perioperative antibiotics are unnecessary.

Numerous studies have shown that employing field preparation sterility for procedures is as effective, if not more effective, than standard sterile prepping or draping. LeBlanc et al. described [34] that following 1504 consecutive carpal tunnel releases performed using WALANT and maintaining field sterility, only 6 superficial infections (0.4%) and no deep infections were reported. In one of our own studies, we demonstrated that among 265 WALANT cases under field sterility, there was a 0% rate of infections at 14 days after surgery and a 0.37% rate of infection at 30 days after surgery [22]. Similar studies that involved more complex procedures

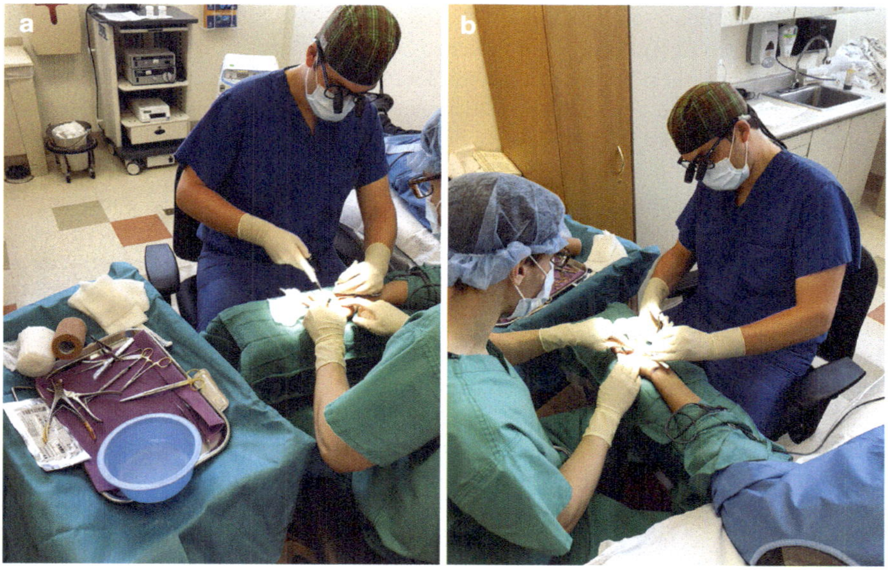

Fig. 16.5 (**a** and **b**): Depiction of performing WALANT for correction of Dupuytren's in an outpatient clinical setting with field preparation sterility

performed using the WALANT with field prep sterility yielded favorable outcomes as well [35–38].

16.3 Advantages of WALANT

The WALANT technique has showcased numerous benefits that include but are not limited to favorable cost savings for the patient and the institution, enhanced patient satisfaction, and limited postoperative pain control. This section delves into the array of advantages associated with WALANT.

16.3.1 Cost

Favorable cost benefits of performing WALANT stem from shorter operative times, decreased utilization of hospital resources and staff, and reduced duration of hospitalization [39, 40]. Patients undergoing WALANT procedures are exempt from the obligation to obtain preoperative evaluation and anesthesia clearance tests due to the avoidance of general anesthesia. Consequently, the expenses associated with standardized preoperative lab tests, medical assessments, and clinic visits are also minimized.

Comparative analyses have demonstrated that WALANT procedures result in significant cost reductions when contrasted with the same procedures performed under general anesthesia or local anesthesia with tourniquet (LAWT), with or without sedation. This cost reduction is attributed to the elimination of preoperative testing, operative room staff, excessive draping, and the infrastructure required for maintaining operating rooms [41, 42]. One study demonstrated that following the analysis of 100 procedures performed under WALANT at a military hospital helped save the military health system $393,100 when compared to the alternative anesthetic methods [25]. Interestingly, another study broke down the cost per minute for all personnel services required for hand cases in the main operating room versus in a procedure room and discovered that the costs in the main OR where general anesthesia or LAWT with sedation were performed were $44 more expensive per minute than those in the procedure room where WALANT was performed [42]. Additionally, Nelson et al. [20] calculated that the cost of performing Dupuytren's surgery under local anesthesia in an ambulatory clinic setting is substantially less expensive than in the main operating room, saving $432.36 per patient compared to fasciectomy under general anesthesia. In the context of a surgeon who performs 25 primary Dupuytren's fasciectomies per year under general anesthesia, the cost savings can reach $10,809.00. However, the actual extent of cost savings in these cases was likely even greater, as the authors did not factor in the expenses related to medications used for managing postoperative nausea and vomiting following general anesthesia, nor did they consider any costs linked to unplanned hospital admissions stemming from complications associated with general anesthesia. For example, one study reported that unplanned overnight hospital admissions following Dupuytren's fasciectomy had occurred in 14% of patients [43].

Due to the cost-effectiveness of WALANT for correction of Dupuytren's contracture, implementing the technique has the potential to make these procedures more accessible to financially disadvantaged patients. For example, in low- and middle-income regions, there exists a significant unmet need for surgical operations due to lack of facilities, proper equipment, and expertise that can be improved with the implementation of WALANT [44, 45]. For example, collaborative efforts between North American hand surgeons and counterparts in Ghana resulted in the establishment of an affordable wide-awake hand surgery facility in Kumasi, Ghana, in 2017. During its first year of operation, this facility performed 360 surgeries at a considerably lower cost, extending the opportunity for local patients to access hand reconstruction who might otherwise not have been able to afford it [46].

16.3.2 Patient Satisfaction and Anxiety

The notion that WALANT surgeries might lead to heightened patient anxiety and discomfort has been a source of concern for many surgeons. However, contrary to this perception, existing literature demonstrates that patient anxiety levels in WALANT cases are equivalent to or lower than those in cases involving general anesthesia or LAWT, with or without sedation. Davison et al. reported that preoperative anxiety levels were significantly lower among WALANT patients than with those who underwent LAWT with sedation for carpal tunnel release [47]. Furthermore, 93% of WALANT-treated patients reported that they would choose WALANT again, a rate on par with patients who received LAWT with sedation. Similarly, other studies have shown that patients undergoing WALANT procedures experienced superior patient comfort scores than those treated with LAWT without sedation or general anesthesia [48–50].

In one study that compared WALANT versus LAWT in 24 patients undergoing bilateral carpal tunnel release, where WALANT was employed for one hand and LAWT for the other, 91.6% of patients reported that WALANT was an easier procedure than expected as compared to 50% with LAWT [51]. Surprisingly, 91.6% of patients even reported finding WALANT easier than a dental procedure [51]. Similarly, Rhee et al.'s study demonstrated that after undergoing WALANT for carpal tunnel release, 94% of patients would choose WALANT again [25].

Experienced surgeons of this technique generally agree that patients experience minimal pain following the initial needle injection, particularly when the injection is administered slowly, when generous volumes of local anesthetic are used, and when sufficient time is given for the local anesthesia to take effect. Furthermore, patients who may be stressed or anxious coming into the new surgical environment tend to adapt quickly once the surgeon explains that there is total numbness and equates the trip to a routine dentist visit.

16.3.3 Postoperative Pain Control

Postoperative pain is equivalent or better controlled with WALANT surgery than with general anesthesia or LAWT, with or without sedation. Miller et al. hypothesized that wide-awake patients undergoing trigger finger release and carpal tunnel release would require increased opioid-based medications to control postprocedural pain compared to patients receiving monitored anesthesia care (MAC) [52]. However, the authors found no difference in total pills consumed between the WALANT and MAC cohorts (3.85 versus 3.95, $P = 0.86$), respectively [52].

Findings from another study indicated that there was no statistically significant difference in opioid usage between patients who underwent WALANT surgery (78 cases; 4.9 pills/cases) versus LAWT with sedation (198 cases; 3.9 pills/case) for carpal tunnel release ($p = 0.22$) [53]. Another study discovered that postoperative pain was statistically lower in the WALANT group in both open cubital tunnel and carpal tunnel surgeries when compared to the other methods of anesthesia such as general versus LAWT, as evidenced by reduced postoperative opioid usage [54]. Furthermore, Dar et al. [55] demonstrated that only a mere 2.1% of WALANT patients sought out opioids from providers, as opposed to 20% of patients who underwent the same procedures under LAWT with sedation.

Furthermore, a notable advantage of WALANT over MAC has recently come to light. In a previously published study [56], pain was effectively managed in 97.9% of WALANT patients without postoperative opioid pain management. The study also described that a significantly higher proportion of MAC patients (19.4%) sought opioid prescriptions from external providers to manage postoperative pain, in comparison to WALANT patients (2.1%) [55]. These findings further suggest that the WALANT technique improves postoperative pain outcomes when compared to those receiving monitored anesthesia care.

16.4 Complications

Complications associated with the WALANT approach are relatively rare or have not been frequently reported. In some instances, patients may experience distress, tremors, or nervousness following the local anesthetic injection. However, only a handful of studies documented vasovagal syncope and "adrenaline rush" following the epinephrine injection [22, 57, 58]. Additionally, in 265 WALANT procedures with up to 22 mg/kg of lidocaine with 1:100,000 epinephrine being administered, no instances of systemic toxicity due to local anesthetic were noted [59]. To mitigate such occurrences, we recommend patients undergo injections while lying down on a stretcher that can be placed in Trendelenburg position in order to increase cerebral blood circulation.

In contrast to the previously held belief that epinephrine induces digital ischemia, as discussed in the introduction, only a few studies have reported instances of digital ischemia [60, 61]. Importantly, these cases were all successfully resolved through the administration of phentolamine. We recommend phentolamine be available in the WALANT procedure room in the event that a contraindicated patient (see below) receives lidocaine with epinephrine. We do not routinely check for finger vascularity at the end of a case, nor perform "rescues" with phentolamine. Phentolamine administration is painful. Rather, we educate the patient that the lidocaine with epinephrine will wear off on average 7 h after administration. We inform the patient not to try to "wake" the finger up with hot water as this could induce burns. If the finger is pale or white the next day, all patients are instructed to present to the office or emergency room for a phentolamine rescue. While this may seem a long duration for ischemia, this has borne out as a risk for digit loss.

As we previously mentioned, there is always a concern among inexperienced WALANT surgeons that epinephrine-induced ischemia may mask the rare ischemic digit after full correction of Dupuytren's contracture with secondary vasospasm of the digital arteries. However, proper WALANT injections for Dupuytren's should not result in an ischemic digit and secondary vasospasm is still able to be diagnosed. In more concerning cases, such as accidental division of the digital arteries, we advocate for immediate microsurgical repair. Microsurgical repair of digital vessels can be performed under WALANT [27].

16.5 Contraindications

There are limited absolute and several relative contraindications for the use of WALANT for the correction of Dupuytren's contracture. To begin with, those with a rare allergy to lidocaine should avoid this approach due to the potential risk [62]. Considering that epinephrine has been associated with heightened adhesion of sickled erythrocytes and the potential to trigger a vaso-occlusive crisis [63], we recommend that patients with sickle cell disease should refrain from undergoing WALANT surgery. In a recent study [56], a WALANT procedure was avoided in a patient with glucose-6-phosphate dehydrogenase deficiency since local anesthetics have been shown to induce hemolysis [64].

Currently, we do not offer WALANT as an option in patients with certain comorbidities. These include those with compromised peripheral circulation, severe preoperative ischemia stemming from a prior vascular injury, or those with a diagnosis of scleroderma, Raynaud disease, Buerger disease, or vasculitis [65]. While concerns have been raised regarding the potential for epinephrine to induce unsafe tachycardia in patients with cardiovascular concerns, it's worth noting that we routinely advise and carry out WALANT procedures in high-risk cardiovascular patients without any reservations or complications. Caution should be advised for patients who exhibit anxiety, are non-cooperative, have active infections, possess a needle phobia, or display abnormal clotting profiles or bleeding disorder [38]. We suggest obtaining a thorough and comprehensive medical history to address the mentioned contraindications before suggesting or performing WALANT for the correction of Dupuytren's contracture.

Lastly, we have several relative contraindications. First, we avoid WALANT in patients who have had relatively recent collagenase injections. We find that this makes the tissue very difficult to dissect within and the more wet environment of WALANT is very unsuitable for this situation. Next, we do not utilize Kirschner wire fixation after obtaining corrections in patients. We worry that this can contribute to prolonged vasospasm. While we do not hesitate to utilize WALANT for severe contractures, multiple digits, and revisions, we are acutely aware of surgical time. The surgeon must be realistic with their surgical skill and operative abilities. Some surgeons are faster than others without compromising quality. And, remember, the patient has to be lying there awake during this time period. They will need to shift positions and occupy themselves. So, if the procedure is to be very long, the anesthetic may be insufficient, and the patient may be uncomfortable. These are situations where WALANT could be theoretically performed but is simply unreasonable and patient care is ultimately compromised.

16.6 Conclusion

The utilization of the wide-awake local anesthesia with no tourniquet approach experienced a substantial surge in the field since its inception. Even though there may be hesitations among less experienced surgeons regarding the implantation of

WALANT for correcting Dupuytren's disease, our aim was to inform the readers regarding our successful outcomes with this approach. With this cost-effective and patient satisfaction approach, we envision more corrections of Dupuytren's to be conducted by this novel technique.

References

1. Al-Qattan MM. Factors in the pathogenesis of Dupuytren's contracture. J Hand Surg Am. 2006;31:1527–34.
2. Burke F, Dias J, Lunn P, Bradley M. Providing care for hand disorders: trauma and elective: the Derby hand unit experience (1989–1990). J Hand Surg Br Eur. 1991;16:13–8.
3. Lalonde DH. Conceptual origins, current practice, and views of wide awake hand surgery. J Hand Surg. 2017;42:886–95.
4. Hanke H. Fingerspitzennekrose nach in lokalanasthesie ausgerfuhrter operation wegen Dupuytrenscher kontractur. Chirurg. 1936;8:684.
5. Kaufman PA. Gangrene following digital nerve block anesthesia: report of a case. Arch Surg. 1941;42:929–38.
6. Lambert G, Snyers J. Gangrene des doigts consécutive à l'anesthesie loco-régionale. Rev Chir. 1933;52:741.
7. Pelner L. Gangrene of the Toc, following local anesthesia with procaine-epinephrine solution; a clinical and experimental study. Anesthesiology. 1942;3:487.
8. De Rougemont J, Carcassonne F. L'anesthesie regionale dans la pratique journaliere des interventions au niveau des doigts. Presse méd. 1933;41:218–20.
9. Sylaidis P, Logan A. Digital blocks with adrenaline: an old dogma refuted. J Hand Surg. 1998;23:17–9.
10. Wilhelmi BJ, Blackwell SJ, Miller J, et al. Epinephrine in digital blocks: revisited. Ann Plast Surg. 1998;41:410–4.
11. Lalonde D, Bell M, Benoit P, et al. A multicenter prospective study of 3,110 consecutive cases of elective epinephrine use in the fingers and hand: the Dalhousie project clinical phase. J Hand Surg Am. 2005;30:1061–7.
12. Lalonde D, Martin A. Epinephrine in local anesthesia in finger and hand surgery: the case for wide-awake anesthesia. JAAOS. 2013;21:443–7.
13. Lalonde D. Minimally invasive anesthesia in wide awake hand surgery. Hand Clin. 2014;30:1–6.
14. Lalonde DH. Wide-awake flexor tendon repair. Plast Reconstr Surg. 2009;123:623–5.
15. Tang JB. Wide-awake primary flexor tendon repair, tenolysis, and tendon transfer. Clin Orthop Surg. 2015;7:275–81.
16. Warrender WJ, Lucasti CJ, Ilyas AM. Wide-awake hand surgery: principles and techniques. JBJS Rev. 2018;6:e8.
17. Hagert E, Lalonde DH. Wide-awake wrist arthroscopy and open TFCC repair. J Wrist Surg. 2012;1:055–60.
18. Müller CT, Christen T, Heidekruger PI, et al. Wide-awake anesthesia no tourniquet trapeziometacarpal joint prosthesis implantation. Plast Reconstr Surg Glob Open. 2018;6
19. Xing SG, Tang JB. Extending applications of local anesthesia without tourniquet to flap harvest and transfer in the hand. Hand Clin. 2019;35:97–102.
20. Nelson R, Higgins A, Conrad J, et al. The wide-awake approach to Dupuytren's disease: fasciectomy under local anesthetic with epinephrine. Hand. 2010;5:117–24.
21. Leblanc MR, Lalonde J, Lalonde DH. A detailed cost and efficiency analysis of performing carpal tunnel surgery in the main operating room versus the ambulatory setting in Canada. Hand. 2007;2:173–8.

22. Avoricani A, Dar Q-A, Levy KH, Koehler SM. WALANT hand surgery: do the AORN guidelines apply? J Surg Orthop Adv. 2021;30:156–60.
23. Tang JB, Gong KT, Xing SG, et al. Wide-awake hand surgery in two centers in China: experience in Nantong and Tianjin with 12,000 patients. Hand Clin. 2019;35:7–12.
24. O'Neill N, Abdall-Razak A, Norton E, et al. Use of wide-awake local anaesthetic no tourniquet (WALANT) in upper limb and hand surgery: a systematic review protocol. Int J Surg Protoc. 2020;20:8–12.
25. Rhee PC, Fischer MM, Rhee LS, et al. Cost savings and patient experiences of a clinic-based, wide-awake hand surgery program at a military medical center: a critical analysis of the first 100 procedures. J Hand Surg Am. 2017;42:e139–47.
26. Conners KM, Kurtzman JS, Koehler SM. Successful use of WALANT in local and regional soft tissue flaps: a case series. Plast Reconstr Surg Glob Open. 2023;11(1):e4756.
27. Wong J, Lin C, Chang N, et al. Digital revascularization and replantation using the wide-awake hand surgery technique. J Hand Surg. 2017;42:621–5.
28. Abell RG, Page IH. The reaction of peripheral blood vessels to angiotonin, renin and other pressor agents. J Exp Med. 1942;75(3):304–14.
29. Alexander ST, Abdullah S, Singh PSGN, Wen APOY, Sapuan J. Coverage of a firecracker blast injury of the right hand with as chest wall flap under wide awake local anaesthesia no tourniquet technique. Cureus. 2021;13(8):e16962.
30. McKee DE, Lalonde DH, Thoma A, et al. Optimal time delay between epinephrine injection and incision to minimize bleeding. Plast Reconstr Surg. 2013;131:811–4.
31. Higgins A, Lalonde DH, Bell M, et al. Avoiding flexor tendon repair rupture with intraoperative total active movement examination. Plast Reconstr Surg. 2010;126:941–5.
32. Bruns K. Postoperative care and review of complications. Int Anesthesiol Clin. 1982;20:27–36.
33. Palazzo M, Strunin L. Anaesthesia and emesis. I: etiology. Can Anaesth Soc J. 1984;31:178–87.
34. LeBlanc MR, Lalonde DH, Thoma A, et al. Is main operating room sterility really necessary in carpal tunnel surgery? A multicenter prospective study of minor procedure room field sterility surgery. Hand. 2011;6:60–3.
35. Arik H, Coskun T, Kose O. Management of spaghetti wrist under WALANT technique. Hand Surg Rehabil. 2021;40:655–9.
36. Huang Y-C, Hsu C-J, Renn J-H, et al. WALANT for distal radius fracture: open reduction with plating fixation via wide-awake local anesthesia with no tourniquet. J Orthop Surg Res. 2018;13:1–11.
37. Moscato L, Laborde A, Kouyoumdjian P, et al. Trapeziometacarpal (TMC) arthroplasty under Wide Awake Local Anesthesia with No Tourniquet (WALANT) versus Local Anesthesia with peripheral nerve blocks (LAPNV): Perioperative pain and early functional results in 30 patients. Hand Surg Rehabil. 2021;40:453–7.
38. Tahir M, Chaudhry EA, Zaffar Z, et al. Fixation of distal radius fractures using wide-awake local anaesthesia with no tourniquet (WALANT) technique: a randomized control trial of a cost-effective and resource-friendly procedure. Bone Joint Res. 2020;9:429–39.
39. Lalonde D, Martin A. Tumescent local anesthesia for hand surgery: improved results, cost effectiveness, and wide-awake patient satisfaction. Arch Plast Surg. 2014;41:312–6.
40. Van Demark Jr RE, Becker HA, Anderson MC, Smith VJ. Wide-awake anesthesia in the in-office procedure room: lessons learned. Hand. 2018;13:481–5.
41. Codding JL, Bhat SB, Ilyas AM. An economic analysis of MAC versus WALANT: a trigger finger release surgery case study. Hand. 2017;12:348–51.
42. Maliha SG, Cohen O, Jacoby A, Sharma S. A cost and efficiency analysis of the WALANT technique for the management of trigger finger in a procedure room of a major city hospital. Plast Reconstr Surg Glob Open. 2019;7
43. Mandal A, Imran D, McKinnell T, Rao G. Unplanned admissions following ambulatory plastic surgery – a retrospective study. Ann R Coll Surg Engl. 2005;87:466.
44. Grimes CE, Bowman KG, Dodgion CM, Lavy CB. Systematic review of barriers to surgical care in low-income and middle-income countries. World J Surg. 2011;35:941–50.

45. Rose J, Weiser TG, Hider P, et al. Estimated need for surgery worldwide based on prevalence of diseases: a modelling strategy for the WHO Global Health Estimate. Lancet Glob Health. 2015;3:S13–20.
46. Behar BJ, Danso OO, Farhat B, et al. Collaboration in outreach: the Kumasi, Ghana, model. Hand Clin. 2019;35:429–34.
47. Davison PG, Cobb T, Lalonde DH. The patient's perspective on carpal tunnel surgery related to the type of anesthesia: a prospective cohort study. Hand. 2013;8:47–53.
48. Abd Hamid MH, Abdullah S, Ahmad AA, et al. A randomized controlled trial comparing wide-awake local anesthesia with no tourniquet (WALANT) to general anesthesia in plating of distal radius fractures with pain and anxiety level perception. Cureus. 2021;13
49. Gunasagaran J, Sean ES, Shivdas S, et al. Perceived comfort during minor hand surgeries with wide awake local anaesthesia no tourniquet (WALANT) versus local anaesthesia (LA)/tourniquet. J Orthop Surg. 2017;25:2309499017739499.
50. Saleh E, Saleh J, Govshievich A, et al. Comparing minor hand procedures performed with or without the use of a tourniquet: a randomized controlled trial. Plast Reconstr Surg Glob Open. 2021;9
51. Ayhan E, Akaslan F. Patients' perspective on carpal tunnel release with WALANT or intravenous regional anesthesia. Plast Reconstr Surg. 2020;145:1197–203.
52. Miller A, Kim N, Ilyas AM. Prospective evaluation of opioid consumption following hand surgery performed wide awake versus with sedation. Hand. 2017;12:606–9.
53. Chapman T, Kim N, Maltenfort M, Ilyas AM. Prospective evaluation of opioid consumption following carpal tunnel release surgery. Hand. 2017;12:39–42.
54. Kang S-W, Park H-M, Park J-K, et al. Open cubital and carpal tunnel release using wide-awake technique: reduction of postoperative pain. J Pain Res. 2019;Volume 12:2725–31.
55. Dar Q-A, Avoricani A, Rompala A, et al. WALANT hand surgery does not require postoperative opioid pain management. Plast Reconstr Surg. 2021;148:121–30.
56. Kurtzman JS, Etcheson JI, Koehler SM. Wide-awake local anesthesia with no tourniquet: an updated review. Plast Reconstr Surg Glob Open. 2021;9
57. Greene BH, Lalonde DH, Seal SK. Incidence of the "adrenaline rush" and vasovagal response with local anesthetic injection. Plast Reconstr Surg Glob Open. 2021;9:e3659.
58. Pires PJ, Moreira LDA, Casas PPDL. Is it safe to use local anesthesia with adrenaline in hand surgery? WALANT technique. Rev Bras Ortop. 2017;52(04):383–9.
59. Lalonde DH, Wong A. Dosage of local anesthesia in wide awake hand surgery. J Hand Surg. 2013;38:2025–8.
60. Abdullah S, Hua LC, Yun LS, et al. A review of 1073 cases of wide-awake-local-anaesthesia-no-tourniquet (WALANT) in finger and hand surgeries in an urban hospital in Malaysia. Cureus. 2021;13
61. Zhang JX, Gray J, Lalonde DH, Carr N. Digital necrosis after lidocaine and epinephrine injection in the flexor tendon sheath without phentolamine rescue. J Hand Surg Am. 2017;42:e119–23.
62. Bina B, Hersh EV, Hilario M, et al. True allergy to amide local anesthetics: a review and case presentation. Anesth Prog. 2018;65:119–23.
63. Thakkar M, Bednarz B. WALANT and sickle cell disease: a cautionary tale. J Plast Reconstr Aesthet Surg. 2021;74:1633–701.
64. Hegedus F, Herb K. Benzocaine-induced methemoglobinemia. Anesth Prog. 2005;52:136–9.
65. Thomson CJ, Lalonde DH, Denkler KA, Feicht AJ. A critical look at the evidence for and against elective epinephrine use in the finger. Plast Reconstr Surg. 2007;119:260–6.

Chapter 17
Cost Assessments and Considerations

Ashley Titan, Yusha Katie Liu, and Robin Kamal

17.1 Introduction

The prevalence of Dupuytren's contracture is known to increase with age [1]. According to the US Census Bureau, the population of older adults is growing [2]. Considering an aging population, with the current prevalence estimated to be at least 5% in the United States [3], the need for Dupuytren's treatments is expected to rise substantially [4].

Given this context, it's crucial to understand the extensive economic implications of Dupuytren's disease. The economic burden of Dupuytren's disease encompasses various facets that extend beyond the direct costs associated with medical interventions. This encompassing burden takes into account the intricate interplay of various factors, even for patients who have not yet undergone medical intervention, but still contend with the profound effects of the disease on their daily lives and ability to work [5–7]. For example, a qualitative study illuminated the pervasive impact of Dupuytren's disease on individuals' day-to-day activities and self-care. Participants

A. Titan
Division of Plastic Surgery, Department of Surgery, Stanford University, Stanford, CA, USA

Y. K. Liu
Division of Plastic Surgery, Department of Surgery, University of Washington, Seattle, WA, USA

R. Kamal (✉)
Department Of Orthopedics, Stanford University, Stanford, CA, USA

M. B. Gottschalk et al. (eds.), *Dupuytren's Disease*,
https://doi.org/10.1007/978-3-031-85873-4_17

reported that the condition affected their capacity to perform daily tasks—like gripping, illustrated by challenges in opening jars—and personal care, with one individual recounting incidents of accidentally poking their eye while cleaning his or her face. Others also reported that it affected their level of confidence and self-image [5].

The purpose of this chapter is to analyze the costs associated with treating Dupuytren's disease. Specifically, this chapter will review the direct, indirect, and intangible costs, while also exploring the current research addressing the cost-effectiveness of various treatments.

17.2 Defining Costs in Healthcare

To gain insight into the economic aspects of managing Dupuytren's disease, it is crucial to first define the distinct categories of costs. Understanding these costs will serve as a foundation for evaluating the cost-effectiveness of different treatment approaches, allowing one to assess not only the financial considerations, but also the impact on health outcomes in tangible terms such as the number of patients successfully treated [8].

17.2.1 Costs

There are three main types of costs that are important to consider when examining patients with Dupuytren's disease: (1) direct, (2) indirect, and (3) intangible costs as it pertains to individuals, facilities/hospitals, and society [8, 9]. Direct medical costs are related to interventions which include the specific billed procedure/surgery, anesthesia, medications, hospitalization, and postoperative follow-up visits, as well as splints and rehabilitation including physical and occupational therapy (PT/OT) [8]. Indirect costs encompass personal costs associated with treatment or disease such as lost productivity due to lost work hours from the disease process resulting in disability as well as due to disability and time off work post-operatively (listed in Table 17.1) [8, 10]. Intangible costs are the impacts of the disease on a patients quality of life. This can be measured through quality-adjusted life years, which is an assigned dollar value to reductions in quality of life. Intangible costs can also include the psychological suffering of patient or family as well as pain associated with the disease process [8, 11].

Table 17.1 Examples of direct, indirect, and intangible costs

Direct costs	Indirect costs	Intangible costs
Splints	Loss of productivity and/or time off work	Quality of life
PT/OT	Need for caregiver	Quality-adjusted life years
Pharmaceuticals (perioperative, inpatient, and outpatient)	Caregiver loss of productivity	Psychological suffering of the patient
Clinic visits		Pain experienced by the patient
Surgery/procedure		Psychological suffering of family
Surgical/procedure supplies		
Operating room costs		
Anesthesia		
Pathology		
Ultrasound guidance		

17.3 Overview of Treatment Modalities and Their Direct Costs

This section will discuss the key factors influencing intervention decisions, types of interventions offered, short- and long-term direct costs associated with different treatment modalities and variations in cost across different regions.

17.3.1 The Decision to Intervene

Intervention for Dupuytren's disease depends on the severity of the disease and patient's preferences. Intervention is often recommended with patients with digital flexion contractures that limit hand function. Flexion contractures can easily be identified with the Hueston tabletop test, whereby the patient places their hand flat on a table and if unable to have their hand fully flat, it is considered a positive test. A 30-degree metacarpophalangeal joint contracture (or any PIP joint contracture) is often cited as a threshold for consideration for intervention [12–15]. Once a decision to intervene has been made there are a variety of treatment modalities including the following: hand/occupational therapy, pharmacotherapy, radiotherapy, collagenase injections, needle aponeurotomy, fasciectomy, and dermofasciectomy. The majority of current research focuses on open fasciectomy, needle aponeurotomy, and collagenase injection.

17.3.2 Open Fasciectomy

Historically, surgeons considered open fasciectomy the gold standard [12]. Open fasciectomies still make up 60.7% of all interventions for Dupuytren's disease [16]. This procedure involves actual excision of disease tissue which can include skin as well as thickened and contracted parts of the palmar fascia. After excision there is release of the contracture which in turn improves finger mobility. Complications from fasciectomy include infection, wound dehiscence and delayed healing, digital neurovascular injuries, tendon injuries, hematoma, and joint stiffness/contracture [17, 18]. Recurrence rate has been found to be 12–40% [19]. For those who have re-intervention, the mean time to reintervention is approximately 0.9 years in one study with the rate for requiring a reintervention being 3% (4 of 116 fingers in which fasciotomies were performed on) [20].

17.3.3 Needle Aponeurotomy

Needle aponeurotomy gained popularity in the 1990s [21, 22]. Needle aponeurotomy makes up at least 10% of all interventions for Dupuytren's disease [16]. This nonsurgical method is a relatively safe and reliable procedure in initial contracture reduction for specific types of cords. With this method a needle is used to puncture and weaken the cord and result in rupture of the cord to facilitate improved finger range of motion. Its reported complications from needle aponeurotomy are generally infrequent, but they can include skin tears, digital nerve injury, and tendon rupture [17, 18]. Recurrence is common after this intervention, occurring in approximately 50% of all patients [19]. On average, the mean time to recurrence for needle aponeurotomy is 1.8 years [20].

17.3.4 Collagenase Clostridium Histolyticum Injection

Collagenase Clostridium histolyticum injection was introduced as a therapeutic option in 2009 [23]. It is an office-based, minimally invasive, nonsurgical option for the treatment of advanced Dupuytren's disease with palpable cords. Collagenase is injected into the affected cord, and within the next several days the treated joint is manipulated to attempt to rupture the cord [23]. Reported complications from collagenase injections are generally infrequent, but they can include skin tears, digital nerve injury, tendon rupture, and allergic reactions to the injected enzyme in the case of collagenase [17, 18]. Collagenase injections make up 22.9% of all interventions performed for Dupuytren's disease. Its recurrence rate is reported to be 10–30% and on average, the mean time to reintervention for is approximately 0.9 years [16, 19, 20]. Of note, the availability of collagenase injections in different countries around the world has fluctuated significantly over the years, largely due to financial constraints related to the high cost of the drug and challenges with negotiating sustainable rates [21, 24]. For example, in the European Union, collagenase was approved in 2011, but subsequently pulled off the market in 2020, due to commercial reasons [25]. Interestingly, US Patent #7,811,560 for Xiaflex is set to expire in July 2028, which may open the doors for generic collagenase formulations. Time will tell how generic options may impact cost and, in turn, affect trends of treatment by surgeons.

17.3.5 Short-Term Direct Cost of Intervention

As of now, existing literature within the United States predominantly centers on comparing the cost of surgical fasciectomy, needle aponeurotomy, and collagenase injection. There are significant direct cost differences between treatments as well as noticeable variation in these costs from different studies. Across all studies, needle aponeurotomy is consistently reported to be the least costly option (Table 17.2). This aligns with its status as an outpatient office procedure, commonly performed using only local anesthetic and large bore needles. Yet, it is difficult to determine from the current published data if fasciectomy and collagenase injection has the greatest initial direct costs as there is incredible variation in their costs in the literature. Specifically, collagenase injections were 2.2- to 8.5-fold more costly than needle aponeurotomy, with surgical fasciectomy falling in between, roughly 1.7- to 6.7-fold more costly than needle aponeurotomy (Table 17.2) [20, 26–29].

17.3.6 Regional Variation in Short-Term Direct Costs

There are significant regional cost differences for these procedures. For instance, Jain et al. performed a retrospective cohort study using a claims database within the United States. They found a substantial difference in the cost of procedures based on geographical region. This study revealed that in the Midwest and Northeast, the average direct cost of fasciectomy was lower than that of a collagenase injection, while the reverse was true in the West and South regions. Despite this, the types of procedures being performed were still similar between regions [27].

Table 17.2 Variations in initial direct cost of therapeutic interventions

	Surgical fasciectomy	Needle aponeurotomy	Collagenase injection
Herrera et al. [26]	$11240	$4657	Not assessed
Leafblad et al. [20]	$5291	$624	$4189
Jain et al. [27]	$3394	$2010	$4453
Drinane et al. [28]	$5576	$1186	$6032

17.3.7 Long-Term Direct Costs

Beyond the initial treatment, understanding the long-term implications is crucial for both clinicians and patients when choosing between various treatment modalities. This consideration is particularly relevant given that Dupuytren's Disease may recur with any of the interventions (Table 17.3).

Camper et al. examined the one-year direct medical costs for patients with Dupuytren's Disease in the US claims database following their interventions. They found that those who underwent collagenase injections had less direct medical costs even at 3 months after intervention compared to costs incurred by patients undergoing fasciectomy. These differences were primarily driven by costs of outpatient surgery associated with fasciectomy and the costs for physician office visits, lab and pathology tests [30].

Adding weight to these findings, Zah et al. performed a retrospective analysis on patients older than 65 years of age with Medicare. Of 37,374 Dupuytren's patients identified, 2911 (7.8%) received collagenase, while 6258 (16.7%) underwent fasciectomy. Although average annual direct costs were greater for those who underwent collagenase injection there was no significant difference in cost for collagenase vs surgery ($7271 versus $6220, respectively, $P = 0.357$) [29]. Zah et al. also investigated annual healthcare-specific costs with patients with commercial insurance using Market Scan data and found that collagenase injection patients had significantly lower annual costs compared to fasciectomy-treated individuals [31].

Notably, the longest study, Leafblad et al., follows patients for 5 years after intervention [20]. They found that the cumulative cost per digit following needle aponeurotomy, collagenase, and surgery at the five-year time point was $1540, $5952, and $5507, respectively. Interestingly, collagenase injection had the highest rate of reintervention at 2 years compared to needle aponeurotomy and surgical fasciectomy (41%, 23%, vs 4%). At 5 years, collagenase injection had comparable reintervention rates to needle aponeurotomy, while fasciectomy had the lowest reintervention rate (51%, 61%, and 4% respectively). Despite collagenase injection having comparable reintervention rates at 5 years to needle aponeurotomy it had the highest cumulative costs over 5 years compared to needle aponeurotomy and fasciectomy [20]. Given that there is only one study to date that follows patients for

Table 17.3 Variations in direct cost of therapeutic interventions

	Duration of follow up	Surgical fasciectomy	Needle aponeurotomy	Collagenase injection
Camper et al. [30]	3 months	$6204	Not assessed	$5038
Zah et al. [31]	1 year	$5800	Not assessed	$3417
Zah et al. [29]	1 year	$6220	Not assessed	$7271
Leafblad et al. [20]	5 years	$5507	$1540	$5952

5 years, more long-term research is needed to obtain a comprehensive grasp of the economic implications of each treatment option, rather than simply looking at costs associated with a single episode of care especially due to the progressive nature of this disease and potential need for multiple interventions.

17.3.8 Other Treatments and Evaluation of Direct Costs

There have been some investigations into other treatments such as radiotherapy to the affected hand [32, 33] and various pharmaceuticals including anti-tumor necrosis factor intra-nodular injection [34, 35]. These interventions are thought to possibly help halt disease progression and alter the type of need for surgical or procedural interventions, just as how rheumatoid arthritis more often requires surgical interventions prior to the use of biologics [36]. However, research exploring their economic viability remains limited, but is needed given the increasing medical research and likely increased utilization of these therapies.

17.4 Indirect Costs of One Treatment

Dupuytren's disease can have a significant impact on productivity, stemming from both the disability caused by the disease itself and any subsequent interventions. These challenges can be measured in terms of indirect costs, encompassing factors such as lost wages and time away from work [10]. Vukicevic et al. compared the indirect costs associated with collagenase injection and fasciectomy in the United States. They found that compared to patients undergoing open fasciectomy, those treated with collagenase injection had lower mean indirect costs. Specifically, the mean indirect was considerably lower in the collagenase compared to the fasciectomy group ($375 vs. $1108; $p = 0.002$). They postulated that this was due to productivity loss and utilization of short-term disability (9.7% vs. 20.2%), as well as fewer days absent from work (average 2.8 vs. 8.1 days) [37].

Though of different monetary value, trends of indirect costs were similar internationally compared to the United States. For instance, Blake et al. found within a cohort from the Netherlands, patients undergoing limited fasciectomy faced an indirect cost of €2638.64 (USD 2849.07) per patient for productivity loss, with a median return to work within 2 weeks. On the other hand, those undergoing percutaneous needle fasciotomy experienced a cost of €180.93 (USD 195.36), with a median return to work occurring within days [38]. These studies suggest that there are greater indirect costs with surgical fasciectomy. Additionally, the cost and cost-effectiveness of surgical fasciectomy needle aponeurotomy, and collagenase injections vary in the international setting as well as in the United States [39–45].

17.5 The Intangible Costs and Cost-Effectiveness Analysis of Dupuytren's Disease

Cost-effectiveness analysis has been widely used in healthcare to measure health outcomes in physical or natural units, such as life years gained or patients successfully treated. For Dupuytren's disease, several studies have examined cost-effectiveness in terms of quality-adjusted life years (QALYs) [4, 33, 35, 46, 47]. Chen et al. evaluated cost-effectiveness based on traditional willingness-to-pay of $50,000 per QALY. Needle aponeurotomy was found to be cost-effective if the currently reported surgical outcomes for the procedure are accurate, with a near 100% rate of success. Collagenase treatment was deemed cost-effective when the medication cost was below $945. In contrast, in this model, open limited fasciectomy was not considered to be cost-effective [46]. In a separate model study with a simulated cohort of 10,000 individuals with recurrent disease, limited fasciectomy was a cost-effective intervention for recurrent high-severity MCP joint contractures, while needle aponeurotomy was a cost-effective treatment for recurrent low-severity MCP joint contractures as well as PIP joint contractures of any severity. Collagenase injection was not found to be cost-effective in recurrent disease [4]. These studies suggest that treatments differ in their cost-effectiveness as well as their impact on quality of life in the short and long term and work absenteeism, emphasizing the importance of individualized treatment strategies guided by disease severity and economic considerations.

17.6 Specific Considerations for Working Individuals

Although Dupuytren's disease is known to commonly affect the elderly population, more than half of the patients with Dupuytren's disease are employed at the time of treatment [5, 33]. A significant proportion of individuals with Dupuytren's disease have reported having limitations at work due to their disease [7, 38, 48]. Patients who suffer from hand conditions and primarily work in manual labor typically need more time off work than those who mainly have desk jobs [38, 49, 50].

A comprehensive analysis of retrospective databases demonstrated considerable financial implications associated with Dupuytren's disease in working adults within the United States, with a difference in overall costs between working adults afflicted with Dupuytren's disease and their counterparts who do not have this condition. Specifically, working individuals with Dupuytren's had higher annual direct medical costs ($5974 vs $3175) compared to their colleagues who do not have Dupuytren's, as well as higher annual indirect costs ($2737 vs $1309) even when adjusted for other medical comorbidities [51]. Those with Dupuytren's also had overall greater healthcare utilization including outpatient, ED services, and even inpatient services. These disparities underscore the increased financial strain borne by individuals grappling with Dupuytren's disease. This significant divergence in indirect costs, which encompasses aspects like lost productivity and absenteeism due to the disease's impact on hand function, elucidates the broader economic ramifications that extend beyond immediate medical expenditures. Prior research has shown that patients do heavily weigh the drawbacks of all procedures including required time off from work as well as the cost of each procedure [52, 53]. This emphasizes that the economic burden of Dupuytren's disease extends beyond straightforward medical costs typically associated with treatment [51].

17.7 Shared Decision-Making and Informed Consent

Involving patients in treatment decisions through shared decision-making not only enhances patient autonomy but also allows them to understand the economic implications of their choices. Surgeons can provide clear information about the costs associated with different treatments, potential complications, and the likelihood of recurrence to optimize these discussions. This approach fosters trust and ensures that patients are making informed decisions aligned with their values and preferences [52, 54].

To illustrate, Kan et al. highlighted that, for patients with Dupuytren's contracture, the recurrence rate and the degree of residual contracture predominantly dictate the selection of treatment [54]. Kane et al. who utilized a mixed methods approach found that patients make unique tradeoffs that are specific to each treatments. Patients who favored needle aponeurotomy and collagenase injection valued the non-invasive nature, efficiency, and shortened recovery time of these treatments. In contrast, those who opted for fasciectomy were more concerned with a lower recurrence rate and anticipated long-term results [52].

The management considerations for Dupuytren's disease are subject to significant variations arising from differing healthcare systems and geographical locations [20, 27, 28, 39–45, 55, 56]. The disparate reimbursement policies across various countries additionally impact both the patient and the healthcare provider, dictating the accessibility and affordability of different treatment options. These variations underscore the importance of a patient-centered approach to treatment decisions, accounting for individual circumstances, preferences, and the nuanced healthcare landscapes in different regions.

17.8 Conclusion

Hand surgeons play a critical role in the management of Dupuytren's disease, not only from a clinical perspective but also from an economic standpoint. As healthcare costs in the United States rise, comprehending the financial ramifications of Dupuytren's disease is essential for practice management and patient counseling. In evaluating the cost-effectiveness of Dupuytren's treatments, it is imperative to consider a multitude of variables that influence cost, such as insurance coverage, practice setting (e.g., Veterans Affairs, academic institutions, private practice), geographical location, and availability of medications and specialized technologies, as well as patient demographics and employment status. Future long-term studies are needed to investigate the healthcare economics and cost-effectiveness of each intervention over the span of an individual patient's lifetime.

References

1. Hindocha S, McGrouther DA, Bayat A. Epidemiological evaluation of Dupuytren's disease incidence and prevalence rates in relation to etiology. Hand. 2009;4(3):256–69. https://doi.org/10.1007/s11552-008-9160-9.
2. Ortman JM, Velkoff VA, Hogan H. An aging nation: the older population in the United States. 2014.
3. Dibenedetti DB, Nguyen D, Zografos L, Ziemiecki R, Zhou X. Prevalence, incidence, and treatments of Dupuytren's disease in the United States: results from a population-based study. Hand. 2011;6(2):149–58. https://doi.org/10.1007/s11552-010-9306-4.
4. Yoon AP, Kane RL, Hutton DW, Chung KC. Cost-effectiveness of recurrent Dupuytren contracture treatment. JAMA Netw Open. 2020;3(10):–e2019861. https://doi.org/10.1001/jamanetworkopen.2020.19861.
5. Wilburn J, McKenna SP, Perry-Hinsley D, Bayat A. The impact of Dupuytren disease on patient activity and quality of life. J Hand Surg Am. 2013;38(6):1209–14. https://doi.org/10.1016/j.jhsa.2013.03.036.
6. Turesson C, Kvist J, Krevers B. Experiences of men living with Dupuytren's disease-consequences of the disease for hand function and daily activities. J Hand Ther. 2020;33(3):386–93. https://doi.org/10.1016/j.jht.2019.04.004.
7. Bainbridge C, Dahlin LB, Szczypa PP, Cappelleri JC, Guérin D, Gerber RA. Current trends in the surgical management of Dupuytren's disease in Europe: an analysis of patient charts. Eur Orthop Traumatol. 2012;3(1):31–41. https://doi.org/10.1007/s12570-012-0092-z.
8. Bozic KJ, Rosenberg AG, Huckman RS, Herndon JH. Economic evaluationin orthopaedics. JBJS. 2003;85:1.
9. Robinson R. Cost-effectiveness analysis. BMJ. 1993;307(6907):793–5. https://doi.org/10.1136/bmj.307.6907.793.
10. Krol M, Brouwer W. How to estimate productivity costs in economic evaluations. PharmacoEconomics. 2014;32(4):335–44. https://doi.org/10.1007/s40273-014-0132-3.
11. Nho SJ, Kymes SM, Callaghan JJ, Felson DT. The burden of hip osteoarthritis in the United States: epidemiologic and economic considerations. J Am Acad Orthop Surg. 2013;21(Suppl 1):S1–6. https://doi.org/10.5435/jaaos-21-07-s1.
12. Rayan GM. Dupuytren disease: anatomy, pathology, presentation, and treatment. JBJS. 2007;89(1):189.
13. Coleman S, Gilpin D, Kaplan FTD, et al. Efficacy and safety of concurrent collagenase clostridium Histolyticum injections for multiple Dupuytren contractures. J Hand Surg Am. 2014;39(1):57–64. https://doi.org/10.1016/j.jhsa.2013.10.002.
14. Grazina R, Teixeira S, Ramos R, Sousa H, Ferreira A, Lemos R. Dupuytren's disease: where do we stand? EFORT Open Rev. 2019;4(2):63–9. https://doi.org/10.1302/2058-5241.4.180021.
15. Schulze SM, Tursi JP. Postapproval clinical experience in the treatment of Dupuytren's contracture with collagenase clostridium Histolyticum (CCH): the first 1,000 days. Hand. 2014;9(4):447–58. https://doi.org/10.1007/s11552-014-9645-7.

16. Gordon AM, Nian PP, Miller C, Schwartz JM, Choueka J. Comparison of patient demographics, utilization trends, and costs of treatment for Dupuytren's disease in the United States from 2012 to 2019. Ann Plast Surg. 2023;91:547. https://doi.org/10.1097/sap.0000000000003665.
17. Boyer MI, Watson JT, Lou J, Manske PR, Gelberman RH, Cai SR. Quantitative variation in vascular endothelial growth factor mRNA expression during early flexor tendon healing: an investigation in a canine model. J Orthop Res. 2001;19(5):869–72. https://doi.org/10.1016/s0736-0266(01)00017-1.
18. Hirase T, Suresh R, Cotton MO, et al. Percutaneous needle fasciotomy versus collagenase injection for Dupuytren's contracture: a systematic review of comparative studies. J Hand Microsurg. 2021;13(3):150–6. https://doi.org/10.1055/s-0040-1721876.
19. Wong CR, Huynh MNQ, Fageeh R, McRae MC. Outcomes of management of recurrent Dupuytren contracture: a systematic review and meta-analysis. Hand. 2022;17(6):1104–13. https://doi.org/10.1177/1558944721994220.
20. Leafblad ND, Wagner E, Wanderman NR, et al. Outcomes and direct costs of needle aponeurotomy, collagenase injection, and fasciectomy in the treatment of Dupuytren contracture. J Hand Surg Am. 2019;44(11):919–27. https://doi.org/10.1016/j.jhsa.2019.07.017.
21. Byström M, Ibsen Sörensen A, Samuelsson K, Fridén JO, Strömberg J. Five-year results of a randomized, controlled trial of collagenase treatment compared with needle fasciotomy for Dupuytren contracture. J Hand Surg Am. 2022;47(3):211–7. https://doi.org/10.1016/j.jhsa.2021.11.019.
22. Foucher G, Medina J, Malizos K. Percutaneous needle fasciotomy in Dupuytren disease. Tech Hand Up Extrem Surg. 2001;5(3):161.
23. Hurst LC, Badalamente MA, Hentz VR, et al. Injectable collagenase clostridium histolyticum for Dupuytren's contracture. N Engl J Med. 2009;361(10):968–79. https://doi.org/10.1056/NEJMoa0810866.
24. Pajardi G, Parolo C, Willbrand S, Hurst L, Grablutz LB. American and European regulations. In: Pajardi G, Badalamente MA, Hurst LC, editors. Collagenase in Dupuytren disease. Springer International Publishing; 2018. p. 119–30.
25. Basso MA, Bernasconi A, Balato G, Cozzolino A, Famiglietti G, Smeraglia F. Clinical results of collagenase treatment for Dupuytren's disease: a case series study with 2-years follow-up. Acta Ortop Bras. 2023;31(spe1):e259218. https://doi.org/10.1590/1413-785220233101e259218.
26. Herrera FA, Benhaim P, Suliman A, Roostaeian J, Azari K, Mitchell S. Cost comparison of open fasciectomy versus percutaneous needle aponeurotomy for treatment of Dupuytren contracture. Ann Plast Surg. 2013;70(4):454. https://doi.org/10.1097/SAP.0b013e31827e531d.
27. Jain A, Tarabishy S, Carter J, Gonzalez G, Herrera FA. Cost analysis and national trends in the treatment of Dupuytren contracture comparing collagenase injection, needle fasciotomy, and open Fasciectomy procedures. Ann Plast Surg. 2021;86(6S):S625. https://doi.org/10.1097/SAP.0000000000002876.
28. Drinane JJ, Gemoets D, Hoftiezer YAJ, Hoehn J, Eberlin KR. Initial treatment choice affects cost-effectiveness and reintervention rates for Dupuytren contracture: a national census among veterans affairs patients. Hand. 2023;18(5):885–90. https://doi.org/10.1177/15589447211072251.
29. Zah V, Stanicic F, Ruby J, Vukicevic D, Hurley D. Real-world medicare healthcare costs of patients with Dupuytren's contracture treated with collagenase or fasciectomy. Plast Reconstr Surg Glob Open. 2022;10(8):e4480. https://doi.org/10.1097/gox.0000000000004480.
30. Camper SB, Divino V, Hurley D, DeKoven M. Cost per episode of care with collagenase clostridium histolyticum versus fasciectomy for Dupuytren contracture: a real-world claims database analysis. J Hand Surg Global Online. 2019;1(2):57–64. https://doi.org/10.1016/j.jhsg.2018.12.005.
31. Zah V, Pelivanovic J, Tatovic S, et al. Healthcare costs and resource use of patients with Dupuytren contracture treated with collagenase clostridium histolyticum or fasciectomy: a propensity matching analysis. Clinicoecon Outcomes Res. 2020;12:635–43. https://doi.org/10.2147/ceor.S269957.

32. Kadhum M, Smock E, Khan A, Fleming A. Radiotherapy in Dupuytren's disease: a systematic review of the evidence. J Hand Surg. 2017;42(7):689–92. https://doi.org/10.1177/1753193417695996.
33. Dritsaki M, Rivero-Arias O, Gray A, Ball C, Nanchahal J. What do we know about managing Dupuytren's disease cost-effectively? BMC Musculoskelet Disord. 2018;19(1):34. https://doi.org/10.1186/s12891-018-1949-2.
34. Nanchahal J, Ball C, Rombach I, et al. Anti-tumour necrosis factor therapy for early-stage Dupuytren's disease (RIDD): a phase 2b, randomised, double-blind, placebo-controlled trial. The Lancet Rheumatology. 2022;4(6):e407–16. https://doi.org/10.1016/S2665-9913(22)00093-5.
35. Dakin H, Rombach I, Dritsaki M, et al. Cost-effectiveness of adalimumab for early-stage Dupuytren's disease : an economic evaluation based on a randomized controlled trial and individual-patient simulation model. Bone Jt Open. 2022;3(11):898–906. https://doi.org/10.1302/2633-1462.311.Bjo-2022-0103.R2.
36. Park JW, Hwang JS, Gong HS. Rheumatoid hand surgery in the era of biologic therapy: a rheumatologist-oriented overview. J Rheum Dis. 2021;28(4):192–201. https://doi.org/10.4078/jrd.2021.28.4.192.
37. Vukicevic D, Tatovic S, Zah V, Hurley D, Imro M. The burden of productivity loss of U.S. commercially insured patients diagnosed with Dupuytren's disease undergoing collagenase versus fasciectomy treatment. Expert Rev Pharmacoecon Outcomes Res. 2021;21(1):127–36. https://doi.org/10.1080/14737167.2020.1770085.
38. Blake SN, Poelstra R, Andrinopoulou ER, et al. Return to work and associated costs after treatment for Dupuytren's disease. Plast Reconstr Surg. 2021;148(3):580–90. https://doi.org/10.1097/prs.0000000000008224.
39. Brazzelli M, Cruickshank M, Tassie E, et al. Collagenase clostridium histolyticum for the treatment of Dupuytren's contracture: systematic review and economic evaluation. Health Technol Assess. 2015;19(90):1–202. https://doi.org/10.3310/hta19900.
40. Sanjuan Cerveró R, Franco Ferrando N, Poquet JJ. Use of resources and costs associated with the treatment of Dupuytren's contracture at an orthopedics and traumatology surgery department in Denia (Spain): collagenase clostridium hystolyticum versus subtotal fasciectomy. BMC Musculoskelet Disord. 2013;14:293. https://doi.org/10.1186/1471-2474-14-293.
41. Povlsen B, Shields AM, Bhabra GS. Resource utilisation associated with single digit Dupuytren's contracture treated with either surgery or injection of collagenase clostridium histolyticum. Hand Surg. 2014;19(2):205–9. https://doi.org/10.1142/s021881041450021x.
42. Mehta S, Belcher HJ. A single-centre cost comparison analysis of collagenase injection versus surgical fasciectomy for Dupuytren's contracture of the hand. J Plast Reconstr Aesthet Surg. 2014;67(3):368–72. https://doi.org/10.1016/j.bjps.2013.12.030.
43. Atroshi I, Strandberg E, Lauritzson A, Ahlgren E, Waldén M. Costs for collagenase injections compared with fasciectomy in the treatment of Dupuytren's contracture: a retrospective cohort study. BMJ Open. 2014;4(1):e004166. https://doi.org/10.1136/bmjopen-2013-004166.
44. De Salas-Cansado M, Cuadros M, Del Cerro M, Arandes JM. Budget impact analysis in Spanish patients with Dupuytren's contracture: fasciectomy vs. collagenase clostridium histolyticum. Chir Main. 2013;32(2):68–73. https://doi.org/10.1016/j.main.2013.02.012.
45. Sefton AK, Smith BJ, Stewart DA. Cost comparison of collagenase clostridium histolyticum and fasciectomy for treatment of Dupuytren's contracture in the Australian health system. J Hand Surg Asian Pac. 2018;23(3):336–41. https://doi.org/10.1142/s2424835518500327.
46. Chen NC, Shauver MJ, Chung KC. Cost-effectiveness of open partial fasciectomy, needle aponeurotomy, and collagenase injection for dupuytren contracture. J Hand Surg Am. 2011;36(11):1826–34. https://doi.org/10.1016/j.jhsa.2011.08.004.
47. Baltzer H, Binhammer PA. Cost-effectiveness in the management of Dupuytren's contracture. Bone Joint J. 2013;95-B(8):1094–100. https://doi.org/10.1302/0301-620x.95b8.31822.

48. Soreide E, Murad MH, Denbeigh JM, et al. Treatment of Dupuytren's contracture: a systematic review. Bone Joint J. 2018;100(9):1138–45. https://doi.org/10.1302/0301-620x.100b9.Bjj-2017-1194.R2.
49. Gustafsson M, Ahlström G. Problems experienced during the first year of an acute traumatic hand injury – a prospective study. J Clin Nurs. 2004;13(8):986–95. https://doi.org/10.1111/j.1365-2702.2004.01019.x.
50. Neutel N, Houpt P, Schuurman AH. Prognostic factors for return to work and resumption of other daily activities after traumatic hand injury. J Hand Surg Eur Vol. 2019;44(2):203–7. https://doi.org/10.1177/1753193418812645.
51. Macaulay D, Ivanova J, Birnbaum H, Sorg R, Skodny P. Direct and indirect costs associated with Dupuytren's contracture. J Med Econ. 2012;15(4):664–71. https://doi.org/10.3111/13696998.2012.670678.
52. Kane RL, Wood SM, Cichocki MN, Chung KC. Evaluating shared decision-making in treatment selection for Dupuytren contracture: a mixed methods approach. Plast Reconstr Surg. 2023;151(2):255e–66e. https://doi.org/10.1097/prs.0000000000009849.
53. Cichocki MN, Chung WT, Kane RL, Chung KC. Dupuytren contracture: using qualitative data to inform a conceptual framework for shared decision-making. J Hand Surg. 2022;48(2):123–30. https://doi.org/10.1177/17531934221133992.
54. Kan HJ, de Bekker-Grob EW, van Marion ES, et al. Patients' preferences for treatment for Dupuytren's disease: a discrete choice experiment. Plast Reconstr Surg. 2016;137(1):165–73. https://doi.org/10.1097/prs.0000000000001878.
55. Mehdiyev T, Maffei D, Müller V, Mair W, Zimmermann RF, Baur EM. Dupuytren disease: a retrospective cohort study comparing collagenase injection and percutaneous needle fasciotomy. Plast Reconstr Surg Glob Open. 2022;10(10):e4604. https://doi.org/10.1097/gox.0000000000004604.
56. Yamamoto M, Yasunaga H, Kakinoki R, et al. The CeCORD-J study on collagenase injection versus aponeurectomy for Dupuytren's contracture compared by hand function and cost effectiveness. Sci Rep. 2022;12(1):9094. https://doi.org/10.1038/s41598-022-12966-z.

Index

M. B. Gottschalk et al. (eds.), *Dupuytren's Disease*,
https://doi.org/10.1007/978-3-031-85873-4

W

X

Z

The manufacturer's authorised representative in the EU is Springer Nature Customer Service Centre GmbH, Europaplatz 3, 69115 Heidelberg, Germany. If you have any concerns regarding our products, please contact ProductSafety@springernature.com

Printed and bound by CPI Group (UK) Ltd, Croydon, CR0 4YY

30/09/2026

02225233-0001